D0095797

BEATING
BRAIN
FOG

BEATING BRAIN FOG

Your 30-day plan to think
FASTER, SHARPER, BETTER

DR SABINA BRENNAN

First published in Great Britain in 2021 by Orion Spring
an imprint of The Orion Publishing Group Ltd
Carmelite House, 50 Victoria Embankment

London EC4Y 0DZ

An Hachette UK Company

5 7 9 10 8 6

Copyright © Dr Sabina Brennan 2021

Illustration on page 63 by Medium69, Jmarchn licensed under the
Creative Commons Attribution-Share Alike 4.0 International license.
All other illustrations sourced and provided by author.

The moral right of Dr Sabina Brennan to be identified as
the author of this work has been asserted in accordance
with the Copyright, Designs and Patents Act of 1988.

All rights reserved. No part of this publication may be reproduced, stored in a
retrieval system, or transmitted in any form or by any means, electronic, mechanical,
photocopying, recording, or otherwise, without the prior permission of both the copyright
owner and the above publisher of this book.

Every effort has been made to ensure that the information in the book
is accurate. The information in this book may not be applicable in each
individual case so it is advised that professional medical advice is obtained
for specific health matters and before changing any medication or dosage.

Neither the publisher nor author accepts any legal responsibility for any
personal injury or other damage or loss arising from the use of the
information in this book. In addition, if you are concerned about
your diet or exercise regime and wish to change them, you
should consult a health practitioner first.

A CIP catalogue record for this book is
available from the British Library.

ISBN (Trade Paperback) 978 1 4091 9772 0
ISBN (eBook) 978 1 4091 9773 7

Typeset by Richard Carr

Printed and bound in Great Britain by Clays Ltd, Elcograf, S.p.A

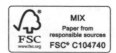

MIX
Paper from
responsible sources
FSC® C104740

www.orionbooks.co.uk

ORION
SPRING

Contents

To David, For Everything
A page to yourself.

Introduction

If you google 'brain fog', as I am sure many of you reading this already have, you will get tens of millions of results in less than a second. But we all know that, when it comes to medical concerns, googling is not the wisest thing to do. It's far better to go directly to a credible source, like the National Health Service (NHS) website, for health information that you can trust. However, if you search for 'brain fog' on the NHS website you will draw a complete blank – 'no results found'. Yet – and I know this from personal experience – if you say that you are experiencing brain fog to friends, colleagues, acquaintances, you will be met with a resounding chorus of others who are also experiencing or have experienced brain fog at some point in their lives.

Brain fog is a collection of symptoms which give rise to loss of mental clarity or foggy thinking. When you have brain fog your symptoms are persistent, occur regularly and interfere with the quality of your life, your relationships and your work. People affected by brain fog experience slowed thinking, problems concentrating and have difficulty focusing their attention. They may also have trouble with remembering, learning new things and can experience language issues such as difficulty finding the right word. Some people affected have difficulties navigating spaces; for example, they may misjudge distances between themselves and objects in their environment, bump into things and might describe themselves as 'clumsy'.

Brain fog is not a diagnosis, disease or a disorder; rather it is a sign or a symptom of an underlying health condition, a side-effect of medication, the result of hormonal changes or the consequence of dietary issues or lifestyle choices.

While clinicians are aware of brain fog, generally speaking, their main concern is the underlying physical or mental health condition, the hormonal imbalance or the deficiencies that can give rise to brain fog symptoms. As you may have experienced if you've gone to see your doctor, they often pay little attention to the brain fog itself. Even when there is an underlying medical condition with multiple symptoms, brain fog can be the most challenging symptom to deal with. Brain fog impacts on your quality of life, can drastically impair your day-to-day functioning and ultimately affects your ability to be human. Brain fog reduces your productivity, your ability to work, run a home or maintain relationships. Even everyday tasks can feel insurmountable when you are struggling to think clearly. But it doesn't have to be that way. This book is brimming with practical tips to help you to minimise the impact that brain fog has on your life and, in many cases, eliminate it completely.

My aim is to translate the academic, scientific and medical evidence on brain fog into easy-to-understand practical information to minimise or eliminate your often debilitating symptoms. I want the millions of people across the globe who experience brain fog to have access to evidence-based advice that they can trust.

Brain fog is a warning that something is amiss, a signal that you need to take action. But brain fog can immobilise you, making it difficult to decide what to buy in the supermarket, let alone decipher complex information or decide which of the millions of pieces of Google advice you can trust.

Having lived through brain fog myself I understand what a challenge it can be. I know what it's like to worry that your symptoms might be the consequence of a life-threatening brain tumour or an early sign of dementia. I understand how difficult it may feel to voice these concerns and how you might want to hide symptoms and hope that no one else notices, for fear that they might think you are no longer capable of doing your job or looking after your kids. I am grateful to everyone who shared their brain fog stories with me. I have changed your names and, in the interests of confidentiality, have blended your stories together.

Even if you have been brave enough to speak to your doctor about brain fog, being met with a response that fails to acknowledge your concerns because you don't have physical symptoms can leave you feeling lost and confused. It's equally frustrating when a doctor, however accurately, suggests that your symptoms might be due to stress, fatigue or 'hormones' but then fails to follow through with tools, treatment or practical advice.

This book gives you both the scientific explanation and an array of potential solutions.

If you feel your doctor is dismissing your concerns, *Beating Brain Fog* will help you to compile the information you need to take to your next appointment, making it more likely that you will be heard and, if appropriate, sent for further investigation and/or treatment. In addition, this book will help you to identify any lifestyle factors underlying your brain fog so that you can take action to better manage it, minimise its impact or banish it completely by incorporating simple brain-healthy habits into your daily life.

With a few notable exceptions, the good news is that brain fog can easily be reversed and eliminated. I firmly believe that knowledge is power and I know that it is possible to change your future for the better when you harness the power of brain health. Read on to learn how to think faster, sharper, better.

How to Use
This Book

The **Knowledge** (Part One) I share in this book will give you the **Power** (Part Two) to **Change** (Part Three) and create a **Future** (Part Four) free from brain fog.

Part One – Knowledge

1 – Know the Enemy: **Brain Fog**

The more you know about brain fog the better armed you will be to beat it. You will learn how to distinguish specific symptoms from each other and link them to brain functions and domains of cognition.[1] Combining this knowledge with the insights that you gain from the self-assessments in this chapter will help you to build a personal brain fog profile and get a clearer understanding of your unique set of symptoms.

2 – Know the Enemy: **Strategy**

This chapter is full of practical strategies to help you to maximise your mental performance while you work through this book. The brain fog profile you create in chapter one will help you to select the most appropriate strategies for your symptoms.

3 – Know Yourself: **Your Brain**

Get to know your brain's structure, workings and communication systems. This knowledge will make it easier for you to understand what is going on in your head in the midst of brain fog and why specific strategies and life choices will help you to minimise your symptoms or banish your brain fog completely.

4 – Know Yourself: **Your Hormones**

Meet your hormones. These chemical messengers are critical to who you are and play a key role in creating your experience of 'self'. If your hormones go out of whack you may no longer feel like 'yourself'. Understanding your hormones, how they work and the role they play in brain fog will help direct you towards appropriate next steps.

5 – Know Yourself: **Your Defences**

Nature is not tidy. The reality is that the systems in your brain and your body interact in complex ways and the smallest imbalance in one system can have knock-on effects that ultimately lead to brain fog. Rather than give an exhaustive overview of your biological processes, this chapter focuses on your immune system and the gut–brain axis because inflammation, infection, pain and issues associated with your gut can contribute to brain fog. This chapter also touches on pharmaceutical treatments that can cause or exacerbate brain fog.

Part Two – Power

6 – **Brain Health**

Brain-healthy habits are the most powerful weapon against brain fog. This chapter explains the scientific principles underlying brain health to help you to understand how brain-healthy habits have the power to prevent, minimise and eliminate brain fog irrespective of underlying causes.

Part Three – Change

Changing your habits in just four aspects of your life will boost your brain health and can dispel brain fog.

7 – Sleep

Experiencing poor quality sleep or insufficient sleep on an ongoing basis can lead to brain fog. Read this chapter for practical tips to improve sleep.

8 – Stress

Stress is not inherently bad but poorly-managed chronic stress can contribute to brain fog. Fortunately there are plenty of pragmatic ways to manage stress.

9 – Exercise

Exercise is critical for a healthy brain. Learn how to build physical and mental fitness to keep brain fog at bay.

10 – Nutrition

What you eat directly affects your brain and how well it functions. You can eat your way to better brain function.

Part Four – Future

11 – 30-day Plan

Learn how to cultivate brain-healthy habits to clear your brain fog and transform your life. There is nothing you can't do once you get your habits right. By performing the daily rituals in this 30-day plan, living a brain-healthy life will become effortless and automatic and your thinking will become, faster, sharper, better.

Epilogue

A brief look at the future of treatment for brain fog.

Part One
Knowledge

If you know the enemy and know
yourself, you need not fear the
result of a hundred battles. If you
know yourself but not the enemy,
for every victory gained you will
also suffer defeat. If you know
neither the enemy nor yourself,
you will succumb in every battle.

The Art of War – Sun Tzu

Know the Enemy: Brain Fog

What is brain fog?

Fog:

(noun) a weather condition in which very small drops of water come together to form a thick cloud, close to the land, sea or ocean, making it difficult to see.

Cambridge English Dictionary

Of course, fog makes it difficult to see. But the experience of fog is so much more than that. Fog creeps. Crawling slowly, it wraps you in a sickly, damp embrace. Fog slows you or stops you in your tracks. Its swirling white veils transform the familiar. Nothing feels the same, nothing feels safe. You see shapes in the shadows but can't make sense of them. Panic rises. Footsteps echo. They sound odd. You can't quite place where they come from. You turn towards a disembodied voice. It feels like a scene from a black and white movie but the soundtrack is muffled and everything is out of focus. You are no longer sure which direction you're facing. Engulfed by the fog. You feel lost.

While dictionaries provide useful definitions, they often tell us little about the actual experience of the phenomenon defined. Just like the definition of fog above, the definition of brain fog below belies the actual experience.

Brain fog:

(noun) a usually temporary state of diminished mental capacity marked by inability to concentrate or to think or reason clearly.

Merriam-Webster Dictionary

My friend Joanne confided in me, 'I feel like I've lost myself to brain fog.' I knew exactly what she meant but I also knew that to anyone who had never experienced brain fog, her words might sound a tad dramatic. I can vouch for the fact that her description is an all too familiar one that echoes the experience of many others who have lived through brain fog, including myself.

Patterns of behaviour define us. We humans are creatures of habit. This predictability shapes our personalities.

'Patsy is always so patient and good natured.'

'John is the life and soul of the party, he's always full of energy.'

'Olive is so witty, she's as sharp as a razor.'

'Amanda is good at everything she turns her hand to.'

Brain fog can disrupt the patterns that shape our personalities; our behaviour becomes less predictable. When we behave out of character we become less recognisable to ourselves and to others. For some, like my friend Joanne, that translates to a feeling of losing themselves. Our relationships can be affected too, as those close to us at home or at work try to make sense of our changed behaviour and abilities, of our new patterns, of who we have become.

Patsy doesn't like who she has become. She says: 'I've no patience anymore. I'm always irritable and cranky.' Amanda feels that she is running on empty and says, 'I just don't have the mental energy for anything more than keeping myself upright.'

Olive's boyfriend told me that Olive, whom he's known since they were both teenagers, has lost her sense of humour. I've known them both since they were kids and agree that this is pretty accurate. It is heartbreaking to watch Olive's dismay at the loss of a part of herself that she loved so much. She was brilliant at banter and you could see she prided herself on her quick wit. 'Without fail, I was the first one with a funny quip. But now I just feel slow. I feel dull. By the time I get the joke the moment has passed.'

For Frances, a woman I used to work with, the experience is more subtle. 'I just feel a bit off. It reminds me of that feeling I get when I sit in my car after someone else has been driving it. The car is still the same but something doesn't feel quite right. Maybe the seat is too far back from the pedals, or it's too low, or reclined too much. Perhaps it's just a small difference in the position of the rear-view mirror or the wing mirrors. It's hard to explain. Everything still works but not quite like it used to. I can still drive my car but it doesn't handle the same way. I feel a little less "in control" than before.'

With brain fog you feel 'off' because your brain is malfunctioning. It is not quite working like it used to. So you don't quite behave like you used to. It's weird because the likelihood is you've never had to think about how your brain works before. It just did. It was seamless. Smooth. Automatic. Now so many things feel effortful. Mechanical. Slow. Off-kilter. That's the brain fog experience.

What are the symptoms of brain fog?

Brain fog is a general term that describes a variety of symptoms. The most common symptoms are: loss of mental clarity, inability to focus or concentrate, problems with learning and remembering, slow thinking, issues with language or word finding and trouble navigating spaces, which many people would describe as clumsiness. If you have ever had brain fog the following will be familiar:

'I just can't think straight.'

'I can't concentrate.'

'My brain feels sluggish.'

'I have trouble recalling what I did yesterday.'

'I really struggle to find the right word.'

'I'm too tired to think.'

'I keep bumping into things.'

Most people will have experienced some, if not all, of these symptoms at some point in their lives. In fact, it is common to have these issues if you have been awake too long, have disrupted sleep, work long hours or are in a stressful situation. Usually the symptoms pass once you catch up on sleep, work reasonable hours or after the stressful situation has been resolved.

Brain fog is different.

In contrast to short-term disruptions, the symptoms of brain fog occur regularly. They interfere with the quality of your life, your relationships and/or your work. Persistent symptoms of this nature are a sign that something is amiss. A signal for you to take action. Reading this book is a fantastic practical first step.

Depending on the context in which they are experienced, the symptoms of brain fog have been referred to as 'baby brain', 'fibro fog', 'chemo brain', 'chemo fog', 'cancer-related cognitive impairment', 'cognitive dysfunction', 'cog fog' and others. Some people describe brain fog as mental fatigue while others count mental fatigue as a symptom of brain fog. Burnout is a recognised medical condition that has many similar symptoms. I use the term brain fog as a 'catch all' to describe the experience of the symptoms, including mental fatigue, irrespective of the context in which they occur or any specific cause or causes.

Brain fog has many shades and affects people in different ways. It can be relatively mild or quite severe, constant or intermittent; it can last for days or persist for years; it can affect just one aspect of cognition or multiple aspects. There is no medical measure for brain fog. That doesn't mean the symptoms aren't real. The impairments to cognitive functioning experienced by people with brain fog have been measured and reported by researchers across a variety of conditions and circumstances and are acknowledged by doctors. The symptoms of brain fog are not only very real, they are often debilitating.

My aim in this chapter is to reassure you that, despite what you are going through, you are neither losing yourself nor your marbles and to remind you that you are not alone. While there are no statistics for the prevalence of brain fog, it is estimated that about 600 million people globally experience cognitive dysfunction, which is a clinical description of brain fog.

This chapter will help you to pinpoint the specific brain functions that are giving you trouble. Once you have done this, it will be far easier to identify and adopt appropriate strategies to improve your symptoms or compensate for lost functioning.

Brain fog is characterised by a range of cognitive symptoms. In psychology, we divide cognitive function into domains. Each domain is responsible for specific behaviours. The key cognitive domains affected in brain fog are:

- Executive function: complex mental processes that you use, for example, to solve problems, make decisions, organise, plan and act towards your goals.
- Attention: when your cognitive resources focus on certain things rather than others, allowing you to selectively process information from your environment.
- Processing speed: the time it takes you to identify, integrate and respond to information in your environment. This impacts on most cognitive functions, including your ability to learn and remember.
- Learning and memory: learning is your ability to acquire new information or a new skill. Memory is complex, but fundamentally it describes your ability to retain information or a representation of a past experience across a period of time. It allows you to retrieve or reactivate the information (e.g. a fact or episode from your life) or the representation (e.g. an image, smell, feeling).
- Language: your ability to understand, express or communicate thoughts, feelings, ideas through the use of sounds, writing or gestures.
- Visuospatial function: your ability to process information through your senses about the relationship between two objects or aspects of a single object, figure or person in three-dimensional space.

Even small impairments to any one of these domains can have considerable impact on your life.

By linking your symptoms to these domains, you will be able to pinpoint which of your neurocognitive abilities are impaired and what interventions or supports will work best for you. Depending on the domain/s affected you may also experience brain fatigue, exhaustion or irritability. If the speed at which information is processed in your brain is slowed then that will have a considerable impact on other aspects of your cognition.

Identifying your brain fog profile

Assessment: Symptom Profile

It's time to get personal. Knowing your own symptoms will take you closer to positive change. Below is a list of common symptoms of brain fog. Place a tick in the box next to any symptoms that you have experienced repeatedly or to the extent that it interfered with your everyday performance or quality of life over the last month. It is important that you only tick where there has been a change in your usual capabilities. We all differ in our abilities. Some of us have always been a bit absent-minded, disorganised or have always had a short attention span. The key, in terms of brain fog, is whether you feel your performance or abilities have deteriorated from your usual baseline.

Executive function

1. ☐ I have difficulty making decisions
2. ☐ I have difficulty solving problems
3. ☐ I have difficulty making plans
4. ☐ I am unusually disorganised or scattered
5. ☐ I have difficulty multi-tasking
6. ☐ I have difficulty thinking clearly, I feel foggy
7. ☐ I feel confused

If you answer yes to any question 1–7 your brain fog profile has an *executive function* component

Attention

8. ☐ I have trouble concentrating
9. ☐ I find it difficult to focus
10. ☐ I have a short attention span

If you answer yes to any question 8–10 your brain fog profile has an *Attentional* component.

Processing speed

11. ☐ I experience slowed thinking
12. ☐ I experience slowed learning
13. ☐ I experience slowed processing of information
14. ☐ I experience slowed reactions
15. ☐ I am slow at completing routine activities

If you answer yes to any question 11–15 your brain fog profile has a *processing speed* component.

Learning and memory

16. ☐ I have trouble with verbal memory (e.g. remembering a conversation)
17. ☐ I have trouble with visual memory (e.g. remembering an image)
18. ☐ I experience forgetfulness
19. ☐ I have problems with short-term memory (e.g. recalling a limited amount of information like a short shopping list after 10–30 seconds)
20. ☐ I have difficulty learning new skills

If you answer yes to any question 16–20 your brain fog profile has a *learning and memory* component.

Language

21. ☐ I have problems expressing thoughts or understanding language
22. ☐ I have difficulty finding the right word

If you answer yes to question 21 or 22 your brain fog profile has a *Language* component.

Visuospatial processing

23. ☐ I have problems navigating spaces (e.g. bumping into things)
24. ☐ I have problems recognising or drawing shapes

If you answer yes to question 23 or 24 your brain fog profile has a *visuospatial processing* component.

Fatigue and Irritability

25. ☐ I experience brain fatigue
26. ☐ I feel mentally exhausted
27. ☐ I experience irritability

If you answer yes to any question 25–27 your brain fog profile has a *fatigue* component.

What is cognition?

Unless you've studied neuroscience or psychology or have a special interest in the brain, it is unlikely that you have an in-depth knowledge of human cognition. For most of my adult life I had nothing more than a vague idea that cognition had something to do with 'knowing'. To be fair, it's not something that pops up in everyday conversation. Which is a little strange, really, when you consider that cognition underlies pretty much everything that we do. It wasn't until I studied psychology at university in my early forties that I began to grasp that cognition refers to 'knowing' in a far broader sense than being in possession of a fact.

Cognition refers to any type of information processing, mental operation or intellectual activity, including: remembering, thinking, attending, reasoning, judging, imagining, learning, perceiving,[2] conceiving and problem-solving. Cognition allows you to reflect on past behaviour, plan future behaviour and override impulsive behaviour. It gives you the ability to imaginatively use knowledge, putting facts, ideas or other information that appear unrelated together to innovate and create novel solutions. Cognition allows you to make sense of and engage with the ever-changing world around you, enabling you to select, receive, transform, store, retrieve and develop information. It also includes the concept of 'self' that Joanne feels that she has lost. Cognition underlies many of your daily activities, so when it is impaired so too is your ability to carry out these activities.

Brain fog profile

Assessment: Brain Fog Profile

Brain fog manifests differently for everyone. One cognitive domain or multiple domains may be affected to varying degrees, from mild to severe.

Use the box below to complete your brain fog profile. Based on your answers above, indicate the domains in which you experience symptoms. Then, on a scale of 1–5, indicate how often you experience these symptoms.

1 = infrequently (less than once a month)
2 = occasionally (at least once a month)
3 = regularly (at least once a week)
4 = often (three or more days per week)
5 = constantly (every day)

Finally, indicate the severity of your symptoms on a scale of 1–5, where 1 is very mild and 5 is very severe.

Domain	Yes / No	Frequency	Severity
Executive function			
Attention			
Processing speed			
Learning and memory			
Language			
Visuospatial processing			
Fatigue			

The symptoms page at the end of this book illustrates how to present this information to your doctor.

You should see a doctor as soon as possible if you:

- have other symptoms that may indicate an underlying medical condition

- notice that your brain fog has started suddenly or worsened significantly
- see no improvement in your symptoms despite making the lifestyle changes in the 30-day plan

Executive function

Executive function is the collective term for several capacities that enable you to exercise self-control, adapt to change and set, manage and maintain goals. Executive function – which you might also hear referred to as executive control or cognitive control – allows you to make plans, think critically, solve problems, make decisions, control your impulses, initiate actions and understand and anticipate the consequences of your own behaviour. Executive function isn't exclusively for intellectual activities; you actually rely heavily on executive function for social, emotional and organisational aspects of your life. For example, if your car breaks down on the way to a job interview and you have issues with emotional control, you may be too upset to think clearly enough to make an alternative plan.

Human beings have a fantastic ability to carry out actions without consciously or actively thinking about them. We call these actions habits or habitual behaviours and it's been reported that more than 40 per cent of our actions each day are habits. This is an energy-efficient way for your brain to operate in the most routine circumstances. For example, every morning my neighbour Tim pours milk on his bran flakes without thinking about it. He's been driving the same route to work for the last ten years so, truth be told, he does it on autopilot. He's never had an accident; he has had a couple of scares but he always managed to pull focus back to the road in time to avoid the cyclist or stop at the red light.

There are plenty of circumstances in which persisting with unthinking, habitual behaviour would be inappropriate, insufficient, impossible or downright dangerous. Thankfully, your executive function gives you the ability to override these automatic, unconscious behaviours so that you can react appropriately to the ever-changing world around you. For example, last week Tim fasted overnight for a blood sugar test.

Next morning, when he opened the fridge to grab the milk carton as he does every day, his executive function stepped in and interrupted his habitual preparation of breakfast with a reminder that he couldn't have anything to eat yet. It also gave him a little nudge to switch off autopilot and consciously drive to the hospital for his appointment rather than take his habitual route to work.

Amanda, a 'stay-at-home' mum, was really surprised to learn how heavily she relies on her executive function. On Wednesday she made a home-cooked meal from scratch for her family (executive function = motivation). She decided what to cook (decision). She got the ingredients together and figured out the order and timings for cooking the various elements (planning and organisation). She kept an eye on the pot bubbling on the stove (monitoring performance). She noticed the dinner sticking to the pot so she reduced the heat and stirred it a little (flexible thinking). While the dinner simmered she did a bit of tidying and sat down to check her social media, while remaining aware that she needed to keep an eye on the cooking and timing of the remaining tasks (task switching). She also managed to resist the temptation to have a biscuit while waiting (inhibition, self-control).

Problems with executive function can have wide-ranging impact affecting even the most mundane tasks. Since developing brain fog, Amanda finds that she has to talk herself through each step of making spaghetti bolognaise, even though she's been making 'spag bol' for her family every week for the last five years.

If your brain fog profile has an executive function component you may notice a drop in your productivity. Depending on the severity of your symptoms, it could impact your job. You may find that your relationships are less harmonious than they once were, especially if your behaviour has become unreliable or you have emotional outbursts. If you've noticed that you are overeating, have gained weight or have become more impulsive, it may well be impairment to your executive functioning that is giving rise to these changes. It's not difficult to see how this could lead you to feel that your quality of life has gone downhill.

Your ability to plan, organise, solve problems and make decisions are guided by three core functions that act together; inhibitory control,[3] working memory[4] and cognitive flexibility.[5]

Inhibitory control

At the most fundamental level, we are creatures of habit who impulsively respond to sensory information in our environment. Everywhere you go your brain is bombarded by incoming sensory information. As you walk along a city street or take public transport, your attention might be caught by an attractive face, an unusual hairstyle, a tattoo, someone's taut abs, a ringing phone, a snippet of conversation or the smell of cigarettes, cologne or body odour. Inhibitory control allows you to override impulsive responses that might be inappropriate in certain contexts.

For social survival it is critical that you keep your impulsive response (verbal or physical) under control. Your brain is acting to protect you when exerting inhibitory control over your impulses. Voicing your unfiltered thoughts or acting on impulse without reflection can got you into trouble. Telling the waiter that his wig 'isn't fooling you or anyone else' won't go down very well. No matter how soft and welcoming the bosom of the woman sitting next to you looks, you cannot lay your head on it to nap on your long train journey.

Inhibitory control allows you to manage your behaviour, emotions, thinking and attention. It enables you to resist the endless pull of sounds, sights, smells and other things that characterise modern life. Inhibition requires effort and this effort places heavy demands on your brain's processing resources. Inhibition not only helps you to regulate your behaviour, it gives you the gift of choice and the means to change your behaviour. Inhibition can be harnessed to help you to break old unhelpful or unhealthy habits and to create new healthy ones. It is something that you can use to help you to eradicate behaviours that cause or contribute to your brain fog.

'Interference control' is a specific type of inhibitory control. Katy and Jim regularly manage to have conversations while cartoons blare on TV and their boys whoop and play. They can do this because interference control allows them to block out irrelevant things (the TV), attend to relevant things (their conversation) and focus on what they choose (the conversation rather than the TV or their kids playing).

'Cognitive control', another subset of inhibitory control, allows you to curb unwanted thoughts, memories and images. This ability is not only helpful for eliminating old habits but is also useful when managing stress, anxiety, depression and traumatic experiences.

'Self-control', which refers to your ability to control your emotions and your behaviours, is yet another subset of inhibitory control. It helps you to resist all kinds of temptation that could be detrimental to your health, your relationships and even to your reputation. For example, you employ inhibitory control when you resist eating a doughnut because you want to attain a healthy weight. Your relationships survive when your capacity for inhibitory control helps you to resist cheating on your spouse with the colleague you get on well with at work. You rely on self-control to behave within socially acceptable norms. Without it you might actually tell your boss that you find him really boring or tell your girlfriend that her bum truly does look big in that dress.

You also exercise self-control when you persist with a task like a college assignment, seeing it through to the end when you would rather be doing something else, like eating buttery toast and chatting with your flatmates.

Gemma has experienced brain fog for a number of years and the thing that she finds most frustrating is the fact that she just can't seem to finish anything anymore. She always considered herself someone who followed actions through to delivery at work and had little time for colleagues who left things half done. So this experience is not only frustrating for Gemma, it goes against a self-defining aspect of herself. She finds this very distressing and guilt-inducing.

Working memory

Working memory and inhibitory control are closely linked. Working memory allows you to hold on to information in your head for a short period of time so that you can manipulate the information to perform a task. Doing maths in your head is commonly used to illustrate working memory and this is something that Amanda finds she can no longer do when brain fog strikes. 'It pains and embarrasses me to have to whip out the calculator on my phone to check I have enough cash on me to pay for the three small items in my basket.'

Working memory is critical for following instructions or keeping track of things or reordering items. It's a bit like a mental notepad. You need it to learn, to reason and to understand.

Working memory is essential for pretty much anything that unfolds over time, because you need to link what happens earlier to what happens now or what comes later. You use working memory to make sense of written or spoken language as you must hold on to information from the start of a sentence or paragraph until the end, when you have the full information required to understand the sense. You even need to employ working memory for something that seems simple, like listening to your friend tell you what happened on her date last night. Brain fog can make it hard to keep track.

Patsy notices this most when she is watching TV. She says she just can't keep all the characters and plotlines clear in her head. 'It became really embarrassing to keep having to ask my seventeen-year-old who was who and what was what. I felt like I was annoying him with my constant questions. So I just don't watch TV with him anymore and I miss that.'

Working memory lets you make comparisons, consider alternatives and make action plans from instructions. It allows you to see relationships and connections between ideas and things. It is critical to creativity and innovation because it lets you break things down into steps or component parts so that you can tease apart elements and recombine them in different ways. Working memory also enables you to bring your memories, previous experience, conceptual knowledge, goals, hopes and desires into the equation when planning and deciding.

Cognitive flexibility

As the name suggests, cognitive flexibility allows you to respond quickly in a flexible way to changed circumstances, different demands or alterations in your environment. As a consequence, you can change directions or plans to avoid risk or to take advantage of unforeseen opportunity. Cognitive flexibility allows you to come up with new solutions by changing how you think about something. Essentially, it supports thinking outside the box, something that Liz was known to be good at. Alas brain fog put paid to that: 'It feels like I've used up all my ideas. Before I could barely keep the lid on my creativity. Brain fog has dried up my creative juices.'

Cognitive flexibility also allows you to think creatively and see things from alternative perspectives and different viewpoints, both spatially (i.e.

'Let's look at this from another angle') and interpersonally (i.e. 'If I were in her shoes'). To achieve this you need to inhibit your previous point of view while you place a different viewpoint on your virtual notepad.

Attention

Brilliant as your brain is, it does not have the capacity to allow you to consciously experience everything going on around you, engage in an unlimited number of actions simultaneously or take in all of the information available to you at any one time. Attention is a finite resource. There is a limit to both the number of things you can focus on and the amount of time that you can stay focused.

Your ability to remain focused is influenced by your interest level and the number of distractions around you. When you concentrate you are selectively applying your attention to a specific object, action, thought or feeling to the exclusion of others. Attention keeps you on task, preventing you from becoming distracted by external (e.g. phone notifications) and internal things (e.g. wandering thoughts).

You can direct your attention to some specific aspect of the world around you, for example, the building you are sketching. Your attention can also be involuntarily captured by something in the environment such as a scent or a car alarm. Internal events such as a rumbling stomach, pain, a memory or a worry can also command your attention. You are more likely to attend to things around you that have meaning for you. For example, lots of your colleagues at work wear perfume or cologne but one in particular stands out for you because it sparks the memory of an illicit kiss at the Christmas party in 2015.

It is perfectly normal for attention levels to wax and wane throughout the day. What is of concern is a notable change in your ability to concentrate or pay attention on an ongoing basis. Many aspects of cognition rely on attention. If any aspect of your attention is impaired you may experience a knock-on effect on other domains of cognition.

There are four core types of attention: selective attention, divided attention, sustained attention and executive attention.

Selective attention

Selective attention allows you to turn your attention and energy to a specific task for a period of time. It allows you to process input from one source of information rather than another. For example, listening to what your spouse is saying and disregarding the competing, and possibly more entertaining, content on the TV.

This ability to attend selectively to a specific aspect of your world allows you to become aware and act on the most urgent. Amanda's ability to hear her baby crying upstairs over the sound of her older kids playing and the noise of the dishwasher allows her to make a decision about whether she needs to go upstairs to attend to her baby or not.

Selective attention happens involuntarily. It involves the inhibition of irrelevant things and the focus of attention on things that are relevant. These two processes occur at the same time. Inhibitory control (see page 21) is similar because it also involves the suppression of distractors. However, inhibitory control doesn't necessarily involve the focusing of attention on things that are relevant. Your brain is constantly taking in information from all of your senses; this selective attention mechanism allows your brain to filter which sounds, which sights and which tasks are most important at any moment in time. Sounds exhausting, doesn't it? Yet when your brain is in good shape this all happens effortlessly.

Unfortunately with brain fog the selective attention system can malfunction, making situations that are usually easy to deal with suddenly challenging. Patsy has worked as a hairdresser for nearly twenty years and has always loved the buzzy atmosphere of the salon with clients chatting and music playing. But lately the noise has become overwhelming to her and she finds herself exhausted by having to concentrate on her clients while feeling distracted by all the other background noise. Her brain has stopped selectively filtering out the noise of the salon for her and having to do this consciously all day to hear what her client is saying is draining her energy and enthusiasm and making her feel irritable.

Divided attention

Divided attention refers to the use of information from multiple sources, attending to more than one task or multiple environmental demands within the same time frame. For example, texting while driving. Divided attention means you will perform less well on each task than you would if you were to attend to one task at a time. This is the reason texting and driving leads to accidents. Don't text and drive.

Sustained attention

Keeping your focus on a specific activity for a prolonged period of time requires sustained attention. Driving, watching a film, reading a book all require sustained attention. Olive has always loved reading. It's her favourite 'me time' activity. However, over the last few months, reading has become a real source of frustration because she just can't seem to focus on what's on the page in front of her. Her thoughts keep wandering and she finds herself having to keep re-reading the same paragraph. She's tried listening to audio books but found that even more frustrating because rewinding on a smart phone is an awful lot more fiddly than turning back a page.

Processing speed

Processing speed refers to the amount of time it takes to perform a cognitive task or certain aspects of a task (e.g. perceive the information, process it, or enact a response). When you scan your wardrobe and choose a suit and shoes that match you are perceiving the contents of your wardrobe, processing this information to find what you are looking for and enacting a response. Processing speed is the amount of time it takes to choose the suit and shoes or to carry out each of the component parts of the process. Essentially, this refers to the pace at which you take in information, make sense of it and begin to respond.

Visual and auditory processing speed respectively refer to how quickly your eyes and ears process seen (e.g. words on a page) or heard (e.g. a news bulletin on the radio) information and relay it to your brain. The pace of your motor response is also an element of processing speed (e.g. how quickly you can turn up the volume on the radio). For Joanne, everything takes longer when she has brain fog. As a consequence, she is finding that she has to stay at work longer just to get through her daily tasks. Having to stay late makes her feel even more tired and stressed, which feeds into a vicious cycle.

Processing speed is a critical element of cognition. Different people process information at a different rate. Pace will also vary depending on the type of information to be processed; for example, words versus figures. When trying to determine whether slowed processing speed is one of your brain fog symptoms, the key is whether your usual pace or pattern has altered or deteriorated.

Learning and memory

Memory is a fundamental cognitive process. Without it your behaviour would be reduced to reflexes. Memory is multi-faceted and different types of memory are processed in different parts of the brain. It can be fleeting, it can be short term or it can be long term. Declarative memory refers to facts and events that can be consciously recalled (declared). Memories may be from episodes from your own life or can be knowledge-based. Remembering your sixth birthday party would be classed as episodic or autobiographical memory. In contrast, remembering that Rome is the capital of Italy is knowledge or fact-based memory, which is also referred to as semantic memory.[6]

Prospective memory refers to remembering to carry out a planned action in the future, such as remembering to take your tablets at 7 p.m. every day or to pick your daughter up from ballet at 3 p.m. on Wednesdays.

Your brain also processes visual, verbal, smell, taste and movement memory. So your sixth birthday memories can be an amalgamation of the smell of fresh cut grass as you played tag with your friends, their shrieks of delight, the distant hum of a lawnmower and the feel of sticky, jammy hands reaching out to tag you.

The memory-making process has three sub-processes: encoding, consolidation and retrieval. During encoding (also called acquisition), when you perceive something in your environment, a new fragile memory trace is formed. The memory trace, prone to deterioration, is gradually stabilised through consolidation processes whereby the new knowledge is embedded within your brain ready for future retrieval.

I know from personal experience how brain fog can impair memory. I've forgotten to pay bills or thought I'd paid bills that I hadn't. One time I even paid my Visa bill twice!

Learning and memory are inextricably linked. Learning is the acquisition of a new skill or knowledge, while memory is the expression of what has been acquired. Learning can occur explicitly (consciously) or implicitly (unconsciously) and can be tested by whether you can freely recall the information learned, whether you need a cue or a hint to 'spark' the memory for the information or whether you recognise the information at all when it is presented to you.

Patsy finds that brain fog makes it really difficult for her to learn how to do new stuff. She says, 'I feel so old. I have to rely on my kids to work anything technical. No matter how many times they tell me how to set up a series link on the TV it just doesn't go in. I have to ask them every time. It's getting so I'd rather not ask because I feel so stupid.'

Language

Language is fundamental to your ability to express yourself through the written or spoken word. Language is also integral to your ability to distinguish and understand sounds and information. Olive says, 'Brain fog makes me feel like my brain isn't connected to my mouth anymore. I can't find the right words to say what I want to.'

Specific sub-domains of language include the ability to name objects, to find the words that you need to communicate, fluency, grammar and syntax (the relationship between words in phrases and sentences). The language domain is critical and includes your ability to comprehend, repeat and express, including finding the right words and names quickly. Language issues in brain fog tend to involve difficulty finding the right word, expressing thoughts or understanding language.

Visuospatial processing

Visuospatial processing refers to your ability to process visual information to understand where objects, including your own body parts, are in space. This ability enables you to determine how near or far objects are from you or from each other. The scene in Irish sitcom *Father Ted* always comes to mind when I think of this, where Father Ted tries to explain the difference between small and far away to Dougal (do look it up on YouTube!). Visuospatial processing also allows you to visualise different images, shapes or scenarios.

Colette recently made the link between her hormonal-related brain fog and what she refers to as 'clumsiness'. 'I've noticed that I get clumsy around the time of my period. I drop things. I bump into furniture in my house that I have no problem navigating my way around at other times of the month. My bed is a particular problem, so much so that when I stub my toe on the corner I know that I'll get my period the next day.'

Interestingly, feeling clumsier was one of the first signs for Amanda each time she became pregnant, to the extent that anytime she dropped her keys or tripped over her own feet her husband joked about another one being on the way.

The ability to process visual and spatial information is essential to understanding and navigating your environment without hurting yourself or getting lost. Most of us would tend to think that bumping into things, dropping things, spilling things or having a poor aim are physical issues but they are in fact cognitive issues.

Fatigue

Fatigue is a signal that you need to rest. Fatigue is a pretty normal temporary response to physical or mental exertion, stress, boredom, insufficient sleep or illness. The tiredness, diminished functioning and impaired mental alertness that characterise fatigue can usually be removed by rest or sleep, just as the hunger signal can be removed by eating. Fatigue cannot be suppressed any more than hunger or thirst can.

John should not ignore the fact that he feels exhausted most of the time – 'I'm just too tired to think.' Fatigue can also be chronic and a sign of an underlying disorder such as chronic fatigue syndrome or anaemia, both of which are discussed in Chapters 7 and 10 respectively.

Finding patterns in the fog

Now that you have a snapshot of your symptoms, it's time to see whether you can detect any patterns to help you to identify triggers, exacerbating factors or causes. The only way to do this is to start keeping a record of your symptoms, when they occur, what you were doing prior to onset and how you were feeling (e.g. stressed, calm). It will also be useful to keep a record of your sleep (quantity and quality) and your exercise levels (none, moderate, over-exercising) and eating habits (irregular, regular, poor diet, healthy diet, undereating, overeating) in the day/s preceding the onset or exacerbation of symptoms.

You can use the table opposite or you can create your own using Excel, a digital calendar or diary. You may already be capturing information on your eating, exercise and sleep habits via apps through your phone, smart watch or fitness tracker. Keep the diary for at least a week, but I recommend keeping it for a month to track your symptoms over a sustained period. If you are serious about beating brain fog, consider keeping a record on an ongoing basis – this will help you to monitor progress, avoid triggers and prevent you from relapsing into old patterns of behaviour.

Identifying patterns can help to assuage some of your fears, reduce frustration and restore a sense of control. Knowing when brain fog is likely to strike will allow you to match your activities to your capabilities at any given time. Recognising your brain fog patterns will also help you to identify and remove triggers. While brain fog can appear out of the blue, with no apparent trigger, there are a number of factors, including poor sleep and stressful events, that reliably bring on or exacerbate brain fog irrespective of its underlying cause.

Once a pattern emerges where, for example, your brain fog is most severe or occurs only after late nights, you can take steps to address the triggers (e.g. eliminate or minimise late nights). Simply knowing that a stressful event has triggered your symptoms can give great comfort and remove frustration because you know that your brain fog will dissipate as soon as the stressful event is resolved. Keeping a record of your symptoms will also restore predictability to your life. Even if you can't eradicate the symptom, simply knowing when it is likely to occur will allow you to plan appropriately and restore some control.

Brain Fog Record

Symptom	Time	Date	Day	Doing	Feeling	Sleep	Exercise	Eating

Summary

- Persistent brain fog symptoms are a sign that something is amiss.
- Brain fog is not a diagnosis, disease or a disorder.
- Brain fog is a general term that describes a variety of symptoms which include:
  o slowed thinking
  o difficulty concentrating
  o problems focusing attention
  o trouble remembering or learning new things
  o language issues
  o fatigue
- The symptoms of brain fog are also referred to as cognitive dysfunction, baby brain, fibro fog, chemo brain, chemo fog, cog fog and cancer-related cognitive impairment.
- Brain fog can be relatively mild or quite severe, constant or intermittent; it can last for days or persist for years; it can affect just one aspect of cognition or multiple aspects.
- Cognition refers to any type of information processing, mental operation or intellectual activity including: perceiving, recognising, remembering, thinking, attending, conceiving, reasoning, judging, imagining, learning and problem-solving.
- Cognition also includes the concept of 'self'.
- Cognition underpins many of your daily activities. When it is impaired by brain fog so too is your ability to carry out these activities.
- Cognition is comprised of a number of cognitive domains which are responsible for specific behaviours or actions.
- The key cognitive domains affected in brain fog are:
  o executive function
  o attention
  o processing speed
  o learning and memory
  o language
  o visuospatial function

- Even small impairments to any of one of these domains can have a considerable impact on your life.
- Depending on the domains affected, you may also experience brain fatigue, exhaustion or irritability.
- Executive function symptoms include: difficulty making decisions, solving problems, making plans, multi-tasking, being organised or thinking clearly.
- Attention symptoms include: trouble concentrating, difficulty focusing and a short attention span.
- Processing speed symptoms include: slowed processing of information, thinking, learning, reactions and completion of routine activities.
- Learning and memory symptoms include: trouble remembering conversations, forgetfulness and trouble learning new skills.
- Language issues tend to involve difficulty finding the right word, expressing thoughts or understanding the spoken or written word.
- Visuospatial problems include: 'clumsiness' and problems recognising shapes.
- Fatigue is a signal that we need to rest.

2

Know the Enemy: Strategy

'He will win who knows when to
fight and when not to fight.'

The Art of War – Sun Tzu

The overarching aim of this book is to empower you to beat brain fog. Having said that, I agree with Sun Tzu, who advises against engaging the enemy until you have a clear advantage. The knowledge you assimilate as a consequence of reading this book will bestow this advantage. In the interim, the strategies below will help you to cope with your current symptoms until you have accumulated the information you need to identify the factors that cause your brain fog and the specific actions to overcome it.

General survival strategies

Focus on what you can do, not on what you can't

It is important to remember that brain fog only affects specific domains of cognitive function. The self-assessments in Chapter 1 will give you a clear picture of your symptoms and the domains affected. While your symptoms may be debilitating, creating your brain fog profile will help you to know your strengths and better match your abilities to the tasks that you need to carry out.

It's frustrating when brain fog prevents you from doing what you had planned. Use your Brain Fog Record to inform your plans in a way that takes account of your fog-related patterns. Always have a plan B so that you can switch activities if needs be. Just because brain fog prevents you from doing one thing, that doesn't mean you have to stop doing everything. Having a flexible plan will help immensely with feelings of frustration and failure.

Know when to persist

Knowing and observing your brain fog in a systematic way will help you to discover when it's wise to persist with activities and when to pause or switch what you're doing. If your brain fog is mild or even moderate, I recommend that you try to persist with the activity that you're struggling with. If you don't challenge your brain, you risk losing further function through disuse. If you injure your leg, depending on the severity or nature of the injury, you might be advised to keep off the leg so as not to exacerbate the injury or you might be told to keep using it to avoid it becoming stiff. Resting will help reduce inflammation and allow the injury to heal, but there is also a cost to this because you may lose muscle tone or ability while your limb is out of action. At a certain point, it becomes necessary to start using the injured limb again. It will be challenging, it may hurt and you may have to relearn how to use it but you must persist in order to retain the ability to walk. The same applies to brain fog and brain function. In a way, you need to carry out a cost–benefit analysis. Rest or disuse will lead to loss of function, so if your symptoms are mild it is probably best to persist to prevent further loss. By contrast, if your symptoms are severe it's best to desist and rest until you notice some improvement, which you will as you work through the programme. In the interim you can adopt some of the domain-specific strategies below to help you to function even with fog.

When brain fog is severe, I recommend that you don't persist with any activity that involves the specific cognitive domain essential for the execution of that very activity. For example, if your executive function is impaired today it doesn't make sense for you to persist with setting up a new filing system or planning that complicated interrail trip across Europe. If feasible, it's far more productive to pause that activity and devote your energy to an activity that doesn't rely heavily on the affected domain. Come back to the original task when the fog has abated, when you feel better able to cope or when you have help (digital or human). If you can't pause the task then it makes sense to call in some troops who are happy to let you tap into their executive function.

It really helps to match tasks to your abilities in the moment. Keep a store of non-urgent, easy, repetitive, non-taxing or manual tasks on your to-do list. When fog strikes you can turn your attention to these. Adopting this approach allows you to remain productive despite brain fog. You will also get a sense of achievement by clearing items off your to-do list.

Know when to resist

It is important to know when your enemy is stronger than you. Resist the temptation to keep on pushing through severe brain fog. When your brain fog is severe, affects multiple domains or is accompanied by exhaustion or mental fatigue, acknowledge that and accept your limits. Stop what you are doing. Take time out. Rest, take a nap or go for a walk.

Know when to relax

When you hit a wall, feel overwhelmed or exhausted, stop what you are doing and take time out to relax. Consider what is truly relaxing for you. Relaxing means different things to different people. Some people find sitting doing nothing wonderfully relaxing. While others, myself included, find it quite stressful to sit and do nothing. I find the physical labour of gardening, decorating or spring cleaning incredibly relaxing but for some that's just hard work. The important thing is to do something that is unaffected by brain fog that makes you feel relaxed.

If you are under pressure or working to a deadline, I advise that you resist the temptation to work late. You, and the work, will benefit from taking the evening off to do something that helps you to shift your focus away from the work challenge. Do something that makes you laugh and have an early night. You may well find that in the morning the solution will come to you. Alternatively, you can just let your brain idle. Don't underestimate the restorative power of daydreaming.

Work with your natural rhythm

Get to know your daily rhythms. Most of us operate within day-to-day routines that have been imposed on us for consistency and social order, such as being at work by 9am. These habitual behaviours can often be out of sync with our natural bodily rhythms. Actively try to pay attention to your body to see if you can tap into its natural rhythm. Are you most alert in the morning? Do you feel sleepy after lunch? Do you have your best ideas in the evening or the morning?

Once you have gathered this intel, combine it with the knowledge that you have of your brain fog patterns and use both to schedule strategically. Diarise tasks that you find more difficult at times of the day when you have the most energy, feel most alert, and are less likely to be tired or distracted. Be realistic about what you can achieve and indeed what others can achieve. Don't place unrealistic demands on yourself or others. Doing so sets the stage for failure and disappointment and will add to stress, which contributes to mental fatigue, making it difficult to think and focus: classic brain fog symptoms.

Make sure to incorporate regular breaks from work. If your job is at a desk, get up from time to time and walk around. Why not add an alarm to your phone or download an app to nudge you to take a break from sitting and prompt you to move every hour or two? Your brain will actually perform better when you stand; this is because sitting for prolonged periods can load to mental fatigue and lack of motion can push your body into sleep mode. Take a break. Go outside for a short walk at lunchtime. Breathe some fresh air. Clear your head, shift your focus from your inner voice to the external world and become aware of the sights and sounds around you.

Don't catastrophise

When brain fog strikes it can be easy to catastrophise, especially if more than one domain is affected. John catastrophised that the mental fatigue and exhaustion that he was experiencing were a sign that he had cancer. Patsy catastrophised that her symptoms were early signs of dementia. She often cried at the thought that her kids would end up having to care for her when they should be enjoying life. Make a conscious effort to put your brain fog in perspective. Remind yourself that brain fog is usually temporary and has multiple causes (many of which you can easily eliminate). It is simply a signal to take action – so start now. Reading this book will help you to identify exactly what actions you need to take.

Exercise

Take aerobic exercise. Becoming aerobically fit will help to strengthen your heart and lungs, allowing your body to pump more blood, containing oxygen and nutrients, to your brain. Chapter 9 discusses the benefits of all types of exercise and offers specific advice for people living with fatigue and pain as a consequence of chronic illness.

Research suggests that regular physical activity protects cognitive function in older adults, young adults and children. Recent research carried out at Columbia University shows that aerobic exercise is good at rescuing lost executive function in adults of all ages. Aerobic exercise will also help you to sleep better, boost your mood and ease depression and anxiety – which is really important since poor sleep, low mood, depression and anxiety all contribute to making your brain fog worse.

Symptom-specific strategies

This section outlines practical strategies for coping with domain-specific symptoms of brain fog. Because these domains are interlinked you will find that some strategies will help across multiple domains.

Executive function

If brain fog makes planning your week, making sound decisions, resolving problems and performing multi-step tasks difficult then you will benefit from adopting some of the strategies below.

Declutter your brain

Get as much information as you can out of your brain and onto paper or electronic devices. Clearing the clutter in your brain will help you to think more clearly and will also free up much-needed cognitive resources. Writing down the stuff that you are struggling with will make some room for you to think more clearly, especially if you are struggling with working memory, which involves manipulating information in your head.

It's easier to manipulate information when you can see it in front of you and can play around with it on the page or computer screen.

Try writing each piece of information on a single bit of paper and physically move it around on a table or on the floor, like you would do if you were planning the seating layout for a wedding. Using working memory to manipulate information in your head is a resource-heavy, taxing cognitive activity. Putting the information on paper and manipulating it physically outside your brain will free up limited cognitive resources, bringing you the same end result but with less strain on your brain.

We often use this outsourcing of cognitive activity when we are tired, stressed, surrounded by distraction or performing under par for other reasons. Cathy is on her way to an interview for a job. She is well prepared but nervous, and really wants this job. She is rehearsing the things she wants to say in her head as she pops into a café to grab a coffee and a croissant. She is early. Standing in line she sees her ex walk past the window with his new girlfriend. She turns her head away sharply. She looks at the prices on the blackboard and the coins in her hand, but she is simply too distracted and stressed to do the maths. In the end she resorts to the equivalent of writing it down, by doing the sums on the calculator on her phone.

Use the notepad or voice memo function on your phone or a small notebook to write down distracting thoughts as they pop into your head. Recording these distracting thoughts will clear them from your brain, allowing you to focus on the task at hand. Recording them also means that you won't forget them if you do need to deal with them at a later stage. When you don't have to 'hold' the information in your brain to manipulate it in working memory, you will free up your limited cognitive resources to carry out the task effectively and efficiently on paper or on an electronic device.

Step back and breathe

It is really important to acknowledge that activities that rely on the executive domain are complex and demanding by their very nature. They require preparation, time, considerable energy and cognitive resources. Take time to think the task through before you begin. If necessary, ask someone to help you with this.

Derick, an experienced architect, says, 'On really bad days I just look at the plans on my desk at work…literally just look at them. I've been doing this job for fifteen years and it's like I've never seen plans before. I can't seem to think clearly enough to make sense of them and this really stresses me out.'

The best thing that Derick can do when this happens is to take a step back and breathe. Feeling overwhelmed by a task or thinking that the task is beyond your capabilities can elicit a stress response which may impair your cognitive abilities further. If you experience moments like this, move your attention away from the task and focus instead on your breathing as it will help to keep you calm and help you to put the task at hand in perspective. Your brain will benefit from the extra oxygen too. Once you are calm again, breaking tasks down into achievable steps can help you to make progress a step at a time without getting stressed or overwhelmed by the work.

Seek support

Call in the support of people that you trust. Identifying your brain fog profile should help you to talk about your experience of brain fog in a tangible way that will make it easier for others to grasp. Explain to family and friends how your experience of brain fog affects your specific functions. Let them know that with their support you can be more like yourself and continue to make decisions and plans. Write out possible solutions to a problem you are facing or list the pros and cons of decisions and thrash them out with someone you trust. Choose wisely – pick someone who you know for sure has your best interests at heart.

Nicky's brain fog made it really hard for her to make decisions. 'I'm not talking life-changing stuff, just deciding what to have for dinner or what to wear to work.' These are hardly decisions that you would approach friends for help with, armed with a list of pros and cons. While her symptoms don't seem too serious they were interfering with her quality of life. Nicky, who lives alone, often felt paralysed standing in front of her wardrobe in the morning. She travels for work a lot and packing became a nightmare; she just felt overwhelmed by figuring out the appropriate clothes for the weather, meetings, travel, evenings, etc.

Eventually she confided in her oldest and best friend Holly. There were tears and Holly even admitted to feeling like that sometimes too. So now Nicky video calls Holly, who helps her pick out clothes and pack. They usually end up having fun in the process and Nicky feels that these calls have actually brought them closer together.

Step by step

When planning your week or your day, or a particular task or activity, use a step-by-step approach, dividing the activity into manageable 'chunks'. Convert your step-by-step plans into a checklist. If you think it would help or give you more confidence, discuss your plans with others to make sure you haven't missed anything.

Get organised

Brain fog can impair organisational skills. Kelly said that within a matter of months she went from being super organised to totally scatter-brained. To combat this, Kelly used whatever supports she could to introduce organised systems to the various aspects of her life.

You can adopt this approach too. Use an online calendar, a diary or wall planner to keep track of obligations. Set up a filing system for important documents. Be disciplined about using whichever method you choose. It might be best to do this when you are symptom free or when your symptoms are mild. Alternatively, get someone to help you to put systems in place. Once the initial organisation is complete, living with brain fog will be smoother and less stressful. It is so worth the initial effort.

Consider setting up automatic payment plans for bills. You could also create a regular weekly schedule. For example, at home you could have a set day for laundry, one for shopping, one for paying bills, etc. Your brain likes regularity and will soon fall into doing these tasks in a habitual way. Building regular habits for regular tasks makes it less likely that you will forget, leave bills unpaid or have to cope with the kids throwing tantrums because their rugby kit hasn't been washed.

Make use of apps and devices like Amazon Echo or Echo Dot. Alexa actually has skills designed to support individuals experiencing issues with executive function.

Be a list maker

Love them or hate them, lists are a fantastic way to free up brain resources, reduce stress and help you to continue to be productive despite living with brain fog. Make checklists for multi-step tasks. Check off each step as you execute it. Save the checklists on your computer or phone. If you prefer, you can make laminated hard copies and use a whiteboard marker to check off each step before wiping it clean for use the next time. Leave checklists in relevant locations around the house or your workplace so you have them to hand when you need them.

Make to-do lists. Use pen and paper, a spreadsheet or apps designed for the purpose. Try to prioritise your list. I routinely enter everything that I have to do into an Excel file which I sort by due date and importance. I find that this allows me to relax into the task at hand without worrying that I should be doing something else. It also prevents me from flitting between tasks, which is an inefficient way to work.

Be realistic about what you can achieve. Try not to be too ambitious. We frequently underestimate how long a task will take. Add a little extra to your estimates to avoid feeling like you are failing or chasing your tail all the time. It can really help to actually measure how long recurring tasks take so that you can make accurate and more realistic estimates.

Cull your lists. Get in the habit of appraising the items on your to do list regularly. Carry over any tasks not done till the next day. If a task constantly gets carried over, ask yourself whether you are avoiding an unpleasant task that needs to be done or whether you have identified a redundant item that you can strike off your list altogether.

Use your friends or lose them

Brain fog can make us behave in out-of-character ways. If your ability to inhibit your speech is impaired you are at risk of saying things that you otherwise might not. Let those close to you know this and ask them to help steer you in the right direction by acting as an external inhibitory controller.

If you notice that you have become more impulsive than you have been in the past, it might be worth recruiting friends and loved ones to help you to wait before responding to a comment that has annoyed or triggered you. If your loved ones have your best interests at heart they will work with you to help you to do that annoying thing that my mother always told me to do as a teen – 'count to ten'. Those ten seconds, or however long it takes to engage your frontal lobes, can help you override the immediate impulsive response that might mean you lose friends or get into trouble.

Alternatively breathe in for a count of four, hold the breath for four, breathe out for four and hold for four. This is called box breathing and can help steady your impulsive tendencies.

If your executive function is impaired, it will help to acknowledge that you really do need to work extra hard to restrain your impulsive responses. Taking extra time, counting or breathing deeply may help you to prevent awkward outcomes or resist temptation if your ability to exercise self-control is currently impaired.

Avoid multi-tasking

Carrying out two or more tasks simultaneously is referred to as multi-tasking. When you check your emails while listening to a presentation, your attentional resource has to be split across the two tasks. As a consequence, you will perform each task more slowly and make more mistakes. This is something that holds true for everyone, not just those of us affected by brain fog, so avoid multi-tasking where possible. When you do something important and potentially dangerous like driving, give it your full attention. Focusing your full attention on driving means no chatting on the phone, no texting, eating or applying make-up.

Strictly speaking, multi-tasking is a myth. When you try to do two tasks at the same time, like talking to someone while texting a friend, you might think that you are multi-tasking, but your brain isn't splitting its attention equally between the two tasks at once. Instead it is rapidly switching back and forth, to texting, then to your friend, then back again. It's no wonder you don't quite 'hear' everything she says when your focus is on the text.

Focus on one thing at a time. Attention is a limited resource. Where possible, avoid spreading it too thinly across multiple tasks. Doing one thing at a time will feel less stressful. You will be less likely to make mistakes and less likely to feel stressed or overwhelmed.

Attention

If you have a short attention span or have trouble concentrating or maintaining focus, take heart. It is possible to train your attention 'muscle'. Read on for tips and strategies.

Turn off autopilot

You're walking to the bus, wondering whether you did definitely unplug the hair straighteners or turn off the grill after you made toast. We've all been there. We blame memory. But the truth may lie elsewhere. It is possible you never 'flicked on' your attention while unplugging the hair straighteners or switching off the grill. Without actively focusing on your own action, the memory is not etched in your brain, so there is nothing to remember. You will just have to go back and check, paying attention to the task this time.

Turn your attention on. Develop a routine in the way you do certain things. For example, always lock up the house or unplug appliances in the same order every time. Store night-time medication with your toothbrush or night clothes or place them on your beside table so you have a visual reminder as you get into bed.

Combat absent-mindedness. It impacts on your ability to remember and it also leaves you more exposed to boredom and low mood. One way to tackle absentmindedness is to learn to focus on the task at hand. Make a point of 'switching on' your attention. This will help you to attend to what you are doing.

Practise mindfulness. Rooted in Buddhist philosophy, mindfulness is when you call attention and focus to the present moment by focusing on breath, body sensation or something in the here and now. Stay in the moment, call your thoughts back from the future or the past. Actively endeavour to concentrate on what you are doing while you are doing it. I often find myself getting my brain to work on something, such as what I might ask my next guest on my podcast or how I might write a section of this book, while I'm physically engaged in another activity, such as cooking, gardening or even eating my dinner. While I might think I am multi-tasking I am missing out on the present, on the joy of being immersed in what I am doing while I am doing it. I doubt I'll ever change completely, and I'm not sure I want to, but I do make an effort to be more focused on what I am doing. Making a conscious effort to be mindful, to be present in the task at hand, will elevate your brain function and give you greater clarity in the experience. Devoting your brain resources to one task at a time will not only make your brain function better, it will boost your mood, make you less irritable, less defensive, happier and more engaged with others. Being mindful can also reduce chronic pain.

Talk yourself through tasks if necessary. Pilots do this. They use self-talk, checklists and talking through their actions with their co-pilot to keep them in the moment. This prevents them from turning their attention off, which is never a good idea when flying an aircraft at 35,000 feet.

Train your attention

You can practise sustained attention, which means holding your concentration on one thing over a long time period. This requires conscious effort and, just as with physical fitness, you need to exercise your focusing skills to keep them in shape. If you haven't been for a run in a while you don't expect to be able to run ten kilometres the first time out. You need to regain your fitness and gradually build up your speed and stamina. The same applies to training your focusing skills – it will be difficult at first, but you will get better at keeping your attention switched on for longer the more you practise it.

Exercise your focusing skills. Gain control over your attention. While listening to a radio talk show, try turning your attention on and off every other minute. Listen intently, allow yourself to drift off, then concentrate again on what is being said. Carry on like this for five to ten minutes. If you practise this technique each day, you'll notice how much the power of your attention can vary. Gradually, your skills at recognising the difference will sharpen and you will be able to tighten your control over your attention.

Remove distractions

It is simply not possible for us to process all of the information our senses take in. Each eye receives approximately 100 megabits of information flow every second. This compares to the fastest broadband connection available. In order not to be overwhelmed by the environment you are in, your brain needs to categorise information as relevant or irrelevant. By doing this it essentially filters out the irrelevant stuff so that you can process the information pertinent to the task.

Help your brain to do this by decluttering your surroundings. Brain fog suppresses your ability to ignore irrelevant or unimportant information. You will find it difficult to focus and are likely to be easily distracted by your surroundings, so removing as many distractions as possible at home or work will help your brain to focus. Reduce noise. Turn off the radio and TV. Go somewhere quiet, away from the kids or colleagues having conversations. If that's not possible, consider noise-cancelling headphones. Listening to soft music on regular headphones can help to drown out distractions too.

Remove visual distractors. If there is constant activity outside it might be better to move away from the window. Even busy home décor can place extra strain on your limited resources. If, for example, you are paying the bills, remove anything from your line of vision that might remind you that you have lots of other things to do, like the laundry or more paperwork. Smells can be distractors too. There's nothing like the smell of toast or coffee to distract you from what you are doing and get you thinking about a coffee break or lunch! If possible, work as far away as you can from both delicious and unpleasant smells.

Attention first – then add meaning

Attention is really the first step in the memory-making process. You need to attend to where you put your keys in order to remember that you put them there. The trick of memory is to make things meaningful. But for this you first need to jump the attention hurdle.

At a party, you join a group and get introduced to three people you've never met before. You say a brief hello, half listen to their names and try to follow the group's conversation, as well as think of what you'd like to say, while also wondering whether you've got food caught between your teeth. Within a few minutes, you are left alone with one of the guests and you can't remember their name or much else about them.

This is a situation in which we will benefit from consciously activating attention. For example, if you want to remember the name of someone you are introduced to, paying attention when you are told it by actively listening is a good start! Be conscious of tuning out distractors like noise in the room and the thoughts running through your head. Next look, really look at the person's face, taking a moment to observe and possibly pick out some memorable feature. Finally, connect the name and the face to some other piece of information that you can associate with them, like their occupation, their dress sense or their personality. Denis the dentist with crooked teeth, or brown-eye Betty with the bad breath. The alliteration will give your memory an extra boost.

Add meaning. Behave as if you are interested in the person's name. Ask questions about it or share a comment: 'Oh, that's an unusual name. Is it French?' or 'What a coincidence, my mum's name was Colette.' You can also add rhyming add-ons to the name to pin on more meaning, perhaps slim Jim, flat-faced Pat, or perfect Pete – you can be as nice or as mean as you like, whatever helps you remember! Make sure you don't say the nickname aloud however, as one of my friends accidentally did to a mutual acquaintance of ours who needless to say is no longer her friend.

You can direct your attention better by repeating the name out loud after hearing it, saying something like, 'Hello, Sarah, how are you?' or asking the person to spell their name for you. Recall the name to yourself after a few minutes and use it in conversation. Nothing polishes a memory like repeated use.

Processing speed

Brain fog can slow our thinking just like a twisted ankle or a bad knee slows our walking speed. You accept that it will take you longer to get from A to B with an injury. You also expect those around you to acknowledge the reality that you will be slower but you will get there in the end. It is important to apply the same principles to brain fog.

Take the time you need

Give yourself permission to take longer than you did in the past to complete the task. Be comforted by the fact that you will get there, it will just take a bit longer. Consider speaking to your employer to seek some tailored adjustments or other reasonable accommodations.[7] You wouldn't think twice about this if you broke your wrist. Allow yourself the time that you need to take in and make sense of the information. Be patient with yourself and ask others to be patient with you. Ask people to speak more slowly, to repeat content or allow you to take notes. Ask colleagues if you can record meetings. Acknowledge that you need time but also remind yourself that you are not daft: your brain simply needs a little more time to process the information than it used to.

Turn off distractions

Turning off distractions like TV, radio and background noise will also help when you are experiencing slowed thinking. It might be an idea to also turn off your mobile phone if you really need to concentrate. Give yourself the best chance possible by avoiding overstimulating environments.

Learning and Memory

Memory is critical to almost everything we do. It can be really unnerving when it fails us during a bout of brain fog, as Elizabeth explains. 'Mid-conversation, I'd start a sentence, then nothing. I'd go completely blank with absolutely no idea what I was going to say. I mean, there was nothing. Just nothing. It wasn't just embarrassing; it was down-right scary.'

Thankfully there are tons of things that you can do to support and supplement your memory. You will be surprised how much difference adopting these strategies can make by freeing up brain space, eradicating unnecessary stress and minimising the impact of brain fog.

Memory aids

We live in such high-tech times that you have probably already used memory aids such as alarms, timers and calendars on your phone or computer. We all use them just to keep pace with the demands of modern life. Making more systematic use of memory aids and apps can really help to support your memory if it is affected.

Make an appointment with yourself and set aside some time to get organised. Choose a time when you are feeling clear headed or when your brain fog symptoms are mild. If that's not possible, enlist the help of friends, family or colleagues to set everything up. Be meticulous about entering all plans, appointments, and deadlines into your digital calendar system. Make sure your calendar syncs with your phone if you're using a calendar on a laptop. Whether it's coffee with a friend, your house insurance renewal date, a doctor's appointment, or a college assignment, enter it into your calendar system as soon as you make the plan. Being disciplined about entering all of your plans and time commitments into your calendar or diary in this way doesn't just act as a memory aid, it can also give you a snapshot of your life to supplement your brain fog record. Depending on what this snapshot reveals, you may identify adjustments that you can make to your schedule to better support you through brain fog.

Include as much detail as you have to hand, such as contact details, meeting locations and directions. I find it really handy to have this information on my phone in case I am running late, have to cancel or get lost. While it might seem like a lot to add to a single diary entry, all it usually involves is simply cutting and pasting the information from the organising email or text message. If the meeting, event or activity is arranged over the phone or in person just get into the habit of typing it directly into the calendar as you make the appointment. I find it helpful to add the purpose of the meeting and names of attendees. I then scan this information as a quick refresher before meetings.

Activate reminders and add one to each entry with an appropriate time scale. Why not set up a regular 'me time' reminder? Carve out some time for yourself to do the things you love, take stock, relax or simply be kind to yourself. Update your address book with full details of your most used contacts. In addition to the basics, why not add the name of your contact's children or their favourite sports team? You could also add a photo for each contact with key information on the photo itself so that when they call you, you have an immediate 'on screen' reminder of their name and any other information you choose to add to the photo. You don't have to do this as one mammoth task. You could simply add the info next time they call.

Take notes. Make use of your phone's notepad and voice record abilities for 'in the moment' note taking. Good old-fashioned memory aids like Post-it notes, to-do lists, notebooks and whiteboards all work perfectly well too.

Keep track. A large wall planner might be helpful if it's hard to keep track of everything that everyone in the family is doing. Ask your kids, partner and loved ones not to assume that you will remember the details of their social calendars and request that they update the planner. Consider asking them to send you reminders during the week of where they will be and, if appropriate, add this to your diary or wall planner. Managing your diary in this way has the added bonus of minimising family misunderstandings and arguments over schedules.

WhatsApp groups are a great way to keep track and can work very well as a reminder system. It's not a replacement for real conversation but it's a quick and easy way to keep up to date and check in when everyone is on the move.

Create a one-drop spot (e.g. a box or drawer) for important stuff in your life that you need (and lose) regularly, such as your keys, glasses, wallet, swipe card, passports, driver's licence, hospital appointment cards, etc. Be strict about putting these items in this designated place and only in this designated place when you come home. Never, ever put them anywhere else. Do this for two or three weeks until it becomes a habit and then you will not only always know where to find these important items but you will benefit from the wonderful side-effects of reduced stress levels and extra time, as you are not chasing round looking for items you have misplaced.

Categorising or chunking information is an invaluable tool for maximising memory performance. Instead of trying to remember a random shopping list (butter, oranges, carrots, cheese, apples, cabbage, grapes and milk) try grouping items together by category – for example, fruit, veg, and dairy. It's much easier to remember three fruits, two veg and three dairy items than a randomly arranged list of eight items. Dividing information into small chunks is particularly useful for numbers with several digits. Remembering the eight-digit number 32145262 is tough but remembering the three numbers 321, 452, and 62 is a lot easier. Mobile phones have lessened the need to memorise telephone numbers but there are still plenty of numbers where 'chunking' can be useful. For example, if you want to commit a long number like your credit card number or one of your many online passwords to memory.

Categorising can also help when you want to retain larger blocks of text from a report or a book, for example. Dispense with non-essential information and break the content into key bullet points. Actively doing this can be far more effective than reading and rereading a paragraph over and over. Reorganising the information that you wish to remember in a way that has meaning for you is also quite effective. Simply putting your own structure or stamp on content can help you to retain it more clearly and for longer.

Get connected

Your brain is a highly organised structure that capitalises on a vast network of interacting connections to get its job done. You can optimise your memory function by involving as many parts of your brain as you can in the memory-making process. Often we focus on repeated verbalisation as a ploy to boost memory. Saying the information you want to remember out loud and listening to yourself repeat it will help to make it stick. We do this in part because that's how we learned to memorise at school.

However, while there is nothing wrong with using just your verbal memory, if you want to increase your chances of being able to retrieve a memory, it is really smart to enrich the memory by switching on as many areas of your brain as possible. You can do this by activating your senses. Each one can play a powerful role in embedding memories, as your brain has the capacity to remember information through any of your five senses; the more senses you involve in making a specific memory, the more routes you have to access that memory. This means that if your verbal memory is performing under par you can still access the memory through other sensory routes. Consciously engaging your senses will help to enrich each memory that you encode. Have you ever been reminded of a romantic moment by the faintest waft of a long-forgotten scent?

As you go about your day, consciously activate your senses, drink in your surroundings and notice the colours. Make it a habit. Listen actively. Are the birds singing? Is the dishwasher humming? What can you smell? Reach out and touch your surroundings, notice how the sofa shifts with your body or how the carpet feels under foot. Next time you take the train or bus, alert your senses at each stop or station. Try to consciously link sensory information about the location with the name of the station. Later in the day, mentally take the same journey again using your senses as a guide.

The memories for each of these senses activate different areas of your brain. If someone is wearing perfume or aftershave, take note of the aroma as you remember his or her name. If a song is playing as you learn a new driving route, think about it when you are driving that route again to help you find your way. Activating more brain areas as you learn can increase the likelihood of remembering something.

Visualisation can be very effective too. Next time you have to remember a shopping list, try 'seeing' these words or items in your mind's eye. Visualisation can be really powerful but if you are out of practice with making mental images it may take a few attempts before it comes easily.

When should I be concerned about my memory?

As we get a little older, experiencing problems with memory can set 'am I getting dementia?' alarm bells ringing. So I want to make it very clear that the memory issues associated with dementia are characteristically different from those experienced with brain fog. However, if you regularly experience any of the following, it is worth chatting to your doctor:

- Disorientation about where you are, or what time of day it is.
- Becoming lost in a place you've been familiar with for years.
- Repeating the same story without realising it.

If you feel concerned about your memory it is always best to err on the side of caution, so arrange a visit to your doctor. Stress can impair memory function so worrying about your memory can actually make your memory worse.

Language

It can be frustrating not being able to find the right word. Colette describes her life with brain fog as one long game of charades.

She laughingly recounts giving her family clues and descriptions as they tried to guess what it is she wanted to say. In contrast, Josie's language difficulties scare her, 'Especially when I find myself saying a word close to the word I want – the word might not have the same meaning but it can be connected in some way. It might begin with the same letter or have some sort of distant association with the word I want but it doesn't have the same meaning. It's not a synonym. I might ask my son to pass me the phone when I mean pass me the remote for the TV. Or I might ask my husband to buy onions when I mean apples.'

Chill and chat

Give yourself permission to take as long as you need and don't be afraid to ask others to give you the time for your thoughts to come together. Everything doesn't have to happen at breakneck speed. Stay socially connected, especially during times of emotional upheaval or when you are feeling anxious or down. Seek the support of those who love you; sometimes simply voicing your fears can give you perspective and may even help you to find solutions.

Try to ban stress at these points of anxiety or emotional difficulty. If you feel the stress welling up, attempt to stay calm, relax, take deep breaths and give your brain the time and the space that it needs to do what you want it to do.

Visuospatial processing

People with brain fog often report feeling 'clumsy'. The last thing you want when you're feeling under par is to add to your woes by breaking things or injuring yourself. Thankfully, some of the strategies already discussed can help with this symptom too.

Slow down, look and listen

Be present. Focusing on what you are doing while you are doing it will help you to notice your surroundings more and avoid banging into things. Activate your attention and consciously look where you are going. Avoid multi-tasking. This is discussed in detail above, but multi-tasking will make you more likely to have an accident.

Take your time. Slowing down will give your brain more time to assess your surroundings and reduce the likelihood that you will misjudge distances. If your reaction times have slowed, slowing your pace a little might help to bring them in sync.

Manage stress. Stress can slow down your processing speed and reaction times and may impair your peripheral vision. You may be focused on what is stressing you rather than your surroundings, to the extent that you miss obstacles or impair your ability to navigate your environment safely.

Fatigue

Extended periods of cognitive activity can bring on mental fatigue. When living with brain fog, the extra effort and time required to carry out complex or even routine cognitive activities can leave you mentally drained. Making decisions can be exhausting for anyone let alone someone affected by brain fog. Several of the strategies already outlined in this chapter will help to minimise mental fatigue, as will the tips below.

Declutter your surroundings

There are lots of really simple practical ways to declutter. Get rid of non-essential items from your work space. Assign a specific place for everything – this will help you to keep things organised without feeling overwhelmed. Clear your desk before leaving work each day. Tidy up immediately after cooking or eating. Make your bed on rising. Tidy up after any task or activity as soon as you complete it. Always put things in their allotted space. For example, if you hang your coat under the stairs or in your wardrobe do that as soon as you come home and don't be tempted to dump it on the sofa or the back of a chair.

Reconsider how you do things

As I mentioned earlier, we are creatures of habit. Sometimes we do things a particular way simply because that's the way we learned to do it or that's the way we've always done it. We never question why. In fact, we often don't even question why we do it at all. Asking yourself whether everything that you do is absolutely necessary or if there are more efficient and effective ways to carry out certain tasks may reveal surprises that could free up time and reduce stress. Really look at what you spend your time on every day and question whether it is essential and if it causes you stress or brings joy.

Explore opportunities to delegate or automate tasks or avoid duplication – this will help to slim down your to-do list. Is there anything you can do to boost efficiency? Is there anything you can do to minimise stress? Chapter 8 will give you plenty of practical ideas on how you might do this.

Know your limits

Be realistic about what you can achieve and factor your brain fog into the equation when making plans and promises. Don't overcommit. Learn to say no. Know yourself.

3

Know Yourself: Your Brain

Look under the bonnet

If my car breaks down, I have to call a mechanic. I know how to drive my car and I know that it needs fuel to run. I also know that I should put oil and water in it occasionally but that only gets done when my husband asks me, 'When was the last time you put oil and water in your car, Sabina?' If I'm honest, he puts the oil and water in for me because I haven't a clue where it should go. There is no point in me even lifting the bonnet because I may as well be looking into a black hole as looking into an engine. I don't ever want to be left stranded so I pay for membership of a breakdown recovery service. If I took the time to learn even the rudiments of how an engine works, I might be able to save time and avoid embarrassment by knowing how to deal with the easy-to-fix common causes of breakdown. I might even look under the bonnet to check the oil and water myself.

Now that I've confessed this I feel quite bad that I've never bothered to learn about something that I depend on and use most days. See where I'm going with this? Isn't it utter madness that most people have little or no knowledge about how their brain works, how to keep it healthy or what to do if it's not running as well as it should? We rely on our brains 24/7 for everything that we do. There is no breakdown recovery for brains; there is no requirement to have an MOT or a service and you can't trade your brain in for a new model. You have got to make the one you have last a lifetime. Living with brain fog brings this into very sharp focus.

This book is filled with tips and advice to help you to get your brain running smoothly again. But first you need to get under its bonnet, get familiar with its parts and learn the basics about how your brain works. When we know how something works it is far easier to pinpoint the problem and take steps to fix it. Don't worry, you don't need to know everything or get bogged down in brain anatomy or physiology. I've kept neuroscientific terminology to a minimum and limited the information here to what you need to know to beat brain fog. Understanding yourself better is an added bonus of getting to know how your brain works.

You'd be forgiven for thinking that your brain is a solid, bland, beige organ because that's how it looks when we see one in a laboratory setting in films and on television. However, it only looks that way because it has been preserved or 'fixed' by freezing or formaldehyde. The living brain is an altogether more delicate, fragile mass, floating in fluid inside your skull. It's pliable, it's pink and it has a softer consistency than the steak you might buy from your local butcher.

Essentially you have a squishy information superhighway inside your skull.

Your jelly-like brain contains billions of interconnected cells called neurons, which 'talk' to each other via trillions of connections using electrical and chemical signals. Your brain is a powerful, vibrant, dynamic processing system that supports everything you do and underlies who you are and how you behave. This is why brain fog has a far-reaching and devastating impact on our lives.

Your brain and your behaviour are inextricably linked. They constantly interact and influence each other. Your brain is not complete nor is it static. It is a work in progress, continually sculpted by your choices, behaviours and life experiences. The inner workings of the brain that can be revealed by modern technology and scientific advancement offer a mere suggestion of the brain's glorious magnificence. There is so much more to learn but for now we know enough to understand that the brain not only influences our behaviour but is also influenced by our behaviour. This is why making changes to your behaviour, lifestyle and choices will help you to beat brain fog.

Your cognitive abilities underlie your behaviour and help you to understand and act in the world. They enable you to learn new stuff such as how to change a spark plug, remember your first kiss, focus your attention, solve problems like figuring out how to turn fifteen pieces of wood from IKEA into a TV unit and communicate, whether that's talking a toddler down from a tantrum or asking your boss for a raise. And this is all in addition to processing gazillions of pieces of incoming information from the world around you. Read on to get the basics of how this amazing three pounds of ever-active tissue within your skull works and communicates with the rest of your body through trillions of connections in your brain.

How does your brain work?

What you carry inside your skull is the most complex biological structure in the known universe. It is constantly changing and updating. Different parts of your brain process different types of information and many types of brain cells work together to help make you who you are. Your brain's pink and squishy consistency belies its ability to control all of your bodily functions and your behaviours, allowing you to breathe, believe, create, feel, fear, hear, imagine, learn, love, play, plan, perceive, read, remember, see, smell, touch, taste, think, talk and walk. I could go on but you get the picture – your brain is integral to everything and it has an amazing capacity to continually adapt to your ever-changing environment. It also controls your response to challenges including disease, stress, injury, ageing or the next level of your favourite video game.

The evolution of the human brain

The human brain emerged successively over millions of years to become the complex organ it is today. An organ that can not only play video games but also conceive, design, build and make money from them. Figure 1 shows the three interconnected components that make up this amazing organ: the reptilian brain (brain stem), the emotional brain (limbic system) and the thinking brain (neocortex).

Working from the inside out, the core, the oldest part of the human brain in evolutionary terms, contains the brain stem. The brain stem, which some people call the reptilian brain, contains the structures that keep us alive. These structures are responsible for critical functions that you don't have to consciously think about, such as breathing, heart rate, blood pressure and digestion. Thanks to TV medical dramas like *ER* and *Casualty*, most of us know that if your brain stem is scuppered then so are you unless you have access to a life support machine.

The reptilian brain also contains structures that produce chemicals called neurotransmitters that influence your mood and play a role in depression and anxiety, which are often associated with brain fog. This evolutionarily old part of the brain includes the tennis ball-like structure at the nape of your neck, called the cerebellum, which controls movement, balance and coordination.

The 'emotional brain', also called the limbic brain, evolved next, emerging in small mammals about 150 million years ago to manage 'fight or flight' circuitry. Structures within this part of the brain are involved in functions that are often affected by brain fog, including learning, memory, emotions, spatial navigation and the unconscious judgements that can strongly influence behaviour. When Patsy struggles to learn new things like how to set a series link on her TV or control her emotions when she catastrophises, it's her limbic brain that is letting her down.

Your 'thinking brain' or neocortex is a relative newcomer in the evolution of the brain. It emerged in primates two or three million years ago. As its name suggests (neo = new and cortex = cover), it is part of the wrinkled outer layer of your brain. The neocortex is responsible for all of the complex functions that we associate with being human, such as our ability to think and use language, the very functions that are affected in brain fog.

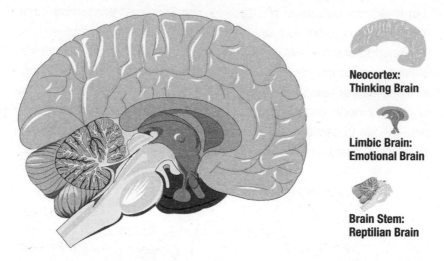

Neocortex:
Thinking Brain

Limbic Brain:
Emotional Brain

Brain Stem:
Reptilian Brain

Figure 1: The three parts of the brain that have evolved over time

The ridges and grooves that give the brain's outer cortex its crinkly appearance are an ingenious exercise in IKEA-style space saving that allows more brain to fit inside your skull. Essentially, the folds enlarge the surface area of the brain, allowing it to accommodate more brain cells and increase capacity for complex behaviour like studying for exams, figuring out your tax returns or calculating how much change you are due in the supermarket.

Your thinking brain is divided into two roughly symmetrical halves called hemispheres. Each hemisphere takes care of one side of your body, but the controls are crossed. This means that the right side of your brain (right hemisphere), takes care of the left side of your body and vice versa.

How is your brain organised?

Each hemisphere of your brain has four lobes (frontal, parietal, temporal and occipital). Broadly speaking, the individual lobes are associated with specific processes and cognitive domains. The lobes depend on information from the world around you to get the job of being you done. The lobes also interact with each other and with the rest of your brain. For example, while the occipital lobes play a key role in vision, it is simply not enough to be able to 'see' something in your environment. You also need to be able to understand what it is you are seeing, so your temporal lobes assign meaning to visual information. When you recognise your mum's face in a photograph or your own child's face in the mêlée of kids pouring out of the school gate it is thanks to the combined workings of your occipital and temporal lobes. Because of this, it's not possible to map a one-to-one relationship between each brain fog symptom and a specific lobe of the brain.

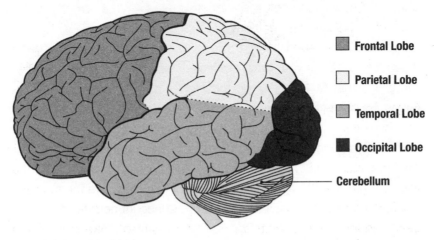

Frontal Lobe

Parietal Lobe

Temporal Lobe

Occipital Lobe

Cerebellum

Figure 2: Lobes of the brain

Your frontal lobes control executive function – that is, all of those complex cognitive abilities that we need to solve problems, make decisions, organise, plan and work towards goals. Many frontal lobe activities define who we are or who we believe ourselves to be. As Gemma said, her inability to finish tasks not only makes her feel frustrated and distressed, it is also at odds with her fundamental sense of who she is so she feels guilty about not seeing tasks through to completion.

If you have an executive function component to your brain fog you can attest to the fact that underperforming frontal lobes can make life really tough. It's not just the big stuff that's affected by frontal lobe failures because executive function is needed for so much of what we do. Without it, it's unlikely that Amanda could make bolognaise for her family. Nicky's frontal lobes let her down when she can't decide what to wear for work or what to pack for her business trips.

Your temporal lobes, which run along the sides of your brain behind your temples, are involved in processing sound, understanding language and producing speech. Your parietal lobes, which sit behind your frontal lobes along the top of your brain, process information coming in from your senses and link this information with existing memories and knowledge, adding meaning to the incoming sensory information.

When you struggle to find a word or remember where you parked your car or left your keys, your frontal, temporal and parietal lobes together with learning and memory structures in your 'emotional' or limbic brain could all be contributing to the problem.

Your occipital lobes are like the eyes in the back of your head because this part of your brain processes visual information. Together with your parietal lobes, your occipital lobes process the type of information critical for moving around and interacting with objects in your environment, like walking around your bedroom without bumping into your bed or pouring just the right amount of milk on your bran flakes.

Emotional underbelly

Your emotional brain sits under the four surface lobes; you'd have to turn the brain upside down to see it. There are three small structures in the limbic brain that you will encounter repeatedly throughout this book because they play a big part in functions that are associated with brain fog, including learning, memory, sleep and stress. They are:

- your hippocampus, which is vital for learning and for making new memories. You actually have two hippocampi, one on either side of the brain, but we tend to mostly talk about this structure in the singular.
- your amygdala, which is involved in the stress response and the processing of emotional memories. You also have two amygdalae, one on either side of the brain, but, the same as with the hippocampi, we tend to mostly talk about this structure in the singular.
- your hypothalamus, which controls the production of many of your body's essential hormones including those that govern sleep and stress.

How does your brain communicate?

The nervous system

The nervous system (NS) is so complex that people have written entire books about it. I've included a diagram (figure 3) of the whole system to give you a sense of how everything fits together, but I will be limiting my discussion to the circled items because I think learning a little about these will help you to understand and beat brain fog. Take a moment to look at the diagram before moving on.

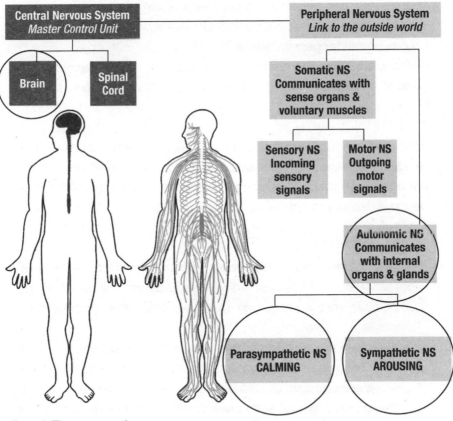

Figure 3: The nervous system

Your autonomic nervous system (see figure 3) plays a key role in managing your internal bodily systems including your stress response, which is of particular relevance to brain fog. Its 'arousing' subsystem is activated by stressors and handles the 'fight or flight' response. The 'calming' subsystem is often referred to as the 'rest and digest' system or the 'feed and breed' system.

Although not shown in figure 3, the enteric nervous system that operates in your gut is also part of the autonomic nervous system. While it is connected to the rest of your nervous system it is a bit of a renegade, operating according to its own rules, and, as a consequence, is sometimes referred to as the second brain. It is connected to and communicates with your brain in a number of ways: via the nervous system using chemical messengers called neurotransmitters; via the endocrine system (see Chapter 4) using chemical messengers called hormones and via your immune system (see Chapter 5) using chemical messengers called cytokines.[8]

What has your gut got to do with brain fog? Well, bacteria in the enteric nervous system also make and communicate using chemical messengers. In fact, the bacteria in your gut secrete and respond to many of the same neurotransmitters released in your brain, including dopamine and serotonin. Since these neurotransmitters have mood-altering properties, your gut bacteria may influence your levels of anxiety or depression which, in turn, can contribute to brain fog, although it's not clear exactly how this occurs.

Talking heads

Like every other part of your body, your brain is made up of cells – approximately 86 billion according to a Brazilian neuroscientist who used a clever method that involved making 'brain soup' to count them. Brain cells are called neurons. Each and every one of these neurons forms an average of seven to ten thousand connections with other neurons. This means there are as many neuronal connections in your brain as there are stars in the Milky Way. Every thought that you have and everything that you do requires precise communication between the neurons in your brain.

As the basic working unit of the brain, the main function of neurons is to transmit information. Every time you stand up out of a chair, decide to eat an ice cream, listen to the radio or recall a funny story, that information is moving along and between neurons through an electro-chemical process. Neurons (see figure 4) have highly specialised pro-jections called dendrites and axons. The dendrites act like receivers, taking information into the cell body. The axons act like communication cables, taking the information away from the cell body. The communi-cation cables allow information to be passed on to neurons in another part of your brain or elsewhere in your body where it can directly act on other types of cells, including muscle and gland cells.

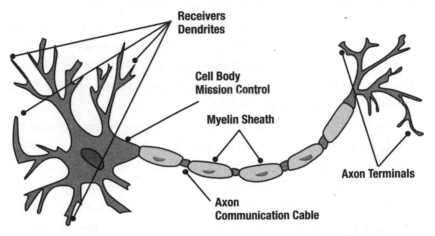

Figure 4: A neuron

Neurons involved in the same function need to communicate with each other in a coordinated way. To do this they form networks. Information travels from one brain cell to the next across a small gap between neurons called a synapse using chemical messengers called neurotransmitters. The neuron that receives the neurotransmitter can further pass it along to other neurons within the network. Each type of neurotransmitter has a particular form that allows it to bind to a receptor on the next neuron in order to produce its effect. It's like a lock and key mechanism – if the neurotransmitter is the right shape it can unlock the response on the next neuron.

Making a habit

Creating brain-healthy habits and eradicating brain fog-inducing habits are critical to beating brain fog. Scientists from MIT have learned a lot about how habits work by recording the activity of rodent brains as they learn how to find a piece of chocolate (reward) in the left side of a T-shaped maze. At the start of the experiment, each rat is placed behind a screen that opens when a loud click (the trigger) is heard. The rats explore the centre aisle of the T-shaped maze, sniffing and scratching as they go. At the top of the T, sometimes the rats turned right and sometimes they turned left. Eventually, most of the rats discovered the chocolate. While the rats appeared to be randomly exploring the maze at their leisure, their brains were a hive of activity, especially in a cluster of neurons called the basal ganglia, located deep beneath the cerebral cortex at the base of the brain.

As the rats moved through the same route hundreds of times they sniffed and explored less and less. The researchers noticed some changes in their brain activity as the rats' behaviour changed with repetition. The rats learned how to navigate the maze quickly and find the chocolate without making wrong turnings and their behaviour became automatic. In parallel, the activity in the rats' brains decreased. The brain activity associated with scratching and sniffing and with deciding to turn right or left ceased. Eventually, even the brain activity associated with memory dampened down. Once the trigger was released, the rats whizzed down the centre aisle and immediately hung a left, going straight for the chocolate. Essentially, the rats had learned a chocolate-finding routine. As the rats performed the routine, the basal ganglia remained active, recalling and acting on patterns and storing habits while activity in the rest of the brain, including the thinking brain, ceased or dampened down. Essentially the rats' brains had chunked together a sequence of actions, converting them into an automated routine and, hey presto, a habit was formed.

In order to conserve energy and save effort your brain adopts the same approach, constantly looking for patterns and routines to turn into habits. This capacity has played a huge role in our evolution. Being able to engage in habitual behaviour – in other words, carry out many tasks on auto pilot – freed up the human brain for innovations and inventions such as harnessing fire for cooking, developing tools, weapons, water systems, the internet, vaccines and so on.

Each of us have hundreds of habitual routines. As I said in Chapter 1, thankfully the brain has a mechanism to interrupt these habits, which allows us to engage in thoughtful behaviour when needed, such as when Tim needed to fast rather than tuck into his habitual bowl of bran flakes. The brain also seems to bookend habitual behaviours with activity. In other words, the brain invests effort at the beginning of a habit looking for a cue (e.g. the loud click), to indicate which routine (e.g. centre aisle then turn left) to use and also at the end of the habit when the reward (chocolate) is attained, to make sure everything went according to plan.

Without habits, the human brain would become overwhelmed with all of the choices and decisions about how to behave and act that need to be made throughout every minute of every day. In fact, people with injury or damage to the basal ganglia become paralysed by basic actions. Even turning on a light switch, opening a door or deciding what to wear can stop them in their tracks.

Speed and flexibility

Electrical conduction gives the brain its speed. Neurons need to send nerve impulses rapidly. Another type of brain cell called glial cells help neurons to do this by wrapping themselves around the communication 'cable' to form an insulation sheath, like the insulation around electrical cables in your home. The white sheath, called myelin, accelerates the conduction of neural signals. In people with multiple sclerosis, these white sheaths become damaged with devastating consequences including brain fog, mobility issues and problems with vision. The portions of the brain that contain myelinated communication cables are commonly referred to as white matter due to the colour of myelin. In contrast, grey matter contains the brain cell bodies.

Electrical transmission gives the brain its speed and the chemical transmission that occurs at the synapse gives the brain its flexibility. Unfortunately, both of these fall victim to brain fog.

Blood brain barrier

Blood vessels are critical to the delivery of oxygen and nutrients to all of the tissues and organs in your body including your brain. The human brain is very vulnerable to toxins. The blood brain barrier (BBB) is a system that acts like border control. The BBB only lets molecules, cells and other matter (e.g. nutrients, water and glucose) with the right credentials through to maintain the conditions critical for optimum brain function. The BBB refuses access to toxins and pathogens[9] such as bacteria and viruses that could cause serious damage or even death. Some research suggests that a faulty BBB lets too many white blood cells into the brains of people with multiple sclerosis. Once across the border, these cells attack the protective sheaths leading to devastating physical and cognitive symptoms.

Hormones

Your nervous system and your endocrine system are responsible for monitoring changes inside and outside your body and responding accordingly. For example, on detecting a drop in the temperature around you, they send signals to cause you to shiver in order to produce heat. Neurotransmitters are the chemical messengers of your nervous system and hormones are the chemical messengers of your endocrine system.

Information in your nervous system is communicated rapidly across synapses so that you can produce instant responses – such as pulling your hand away from a hot flame. In contrast, the overall moods and states that we experience, such as pleasure or depression, depend on hormonal neurons that project their communication cables much more widely. The effects of hormonal neurons take longer to become established in the brain but last longer than those of neurotransmitters. Your nervous system works in tandem with your hormone-producing endocrine system to communicate with the other systems in your body.

Hormonal neurons are concentrated mainly in the brain stem (reptilian brain) and limbic brain (emotional brain). Because they project their communication cables into large areas of the brain they can exert a wide influence. Just one hormonal neuron can influence over 100,000 others. This is because they secrete into the space outside brain cells rather than into the minuscule gap between neurons, which by the way is between 20 and 40 nanometres wide. To put that in perspective, the edge of a sheet of paper that gives you a paper cut is about 100,000 nanometres wide.

Balance

To experience good health free from brain fog, it is critical that optimal conditions are maintained throughout your brain and your body. The many processes by which the body keeps its internal environment in balance are collectively called homeostasis. This is essential to life, ensuring that body temperature, blood pressure, blood sugar levels, oxygen levels etc., are kept within an appropriate range or at a specific set-point. The major biological systems (e.g. respiratory, cardiovascular, nervous, endocrine) in your body work together to ensure homeostasis is maintained. The endocrine system is particularly important because hormones regulate the activity of the body's cells.

Internal and external factors, such as heat, illness, food or fear, can disrupt this critical internal balance. For example, when you eat cake your blood sugar will go up, or if you take a walk on a hot day your internal body temperature will stray from its set-point. Your body has the ability to detect these changes and employ negative feedback loops to oppose these changes and maintain homeostasis. For example, if your body temperature gets too high while you walk in the heat, negative feedback will work to bring it back to its set-point of 37°C. Sensors in your skin and your brain tell the hypothalamus that your internal body temperature has exceeded its optimum set-point; in response, mechanisms in your body are activated to restore optimal conditions. In order to bring your internal body temperature down your blood vessels will dilate, increasing blood flow to your skin which will speed up heat loss. You will also begin to sweat, bringing your body temperature down as the evaporating sweat helps you to cool off. Losing heat to the environment in this way allows your internal body temperature to return to normal.

The microbes[10] in your gut also sustain homeostasis by maintaining a core group of gut microbes. After you eat a meal, new species might appear but between meals your core microbiota[11] will return.

When things go out of balance, deviating from homeostasis, brain fog can be the result. Unfortunately in this instance there is no automatic fallback system to return to homeostasis. Diabetes, which is associated with brain fog, is the result of a broken feedback loop involving the hormone insulin. Throughout this book, you will see that time and again

internal imbalance or runaway reactions due to failed feedback mechanisms contribute to brain fog either directly or indirectly.

There you have it, that's how your brain communicates with itself
and with the rest of your body: information moves from receivers to
the cell body (mission control) and along the communication cables
from one neuron to another. In this way, the billions of neurons inside
your body form trillions of connections between them and the signals
that buzz through these networks in your brain, modulated by your
hormones and influenced by what you do and what you eat, support
you to do what you do and be who you are.

4

Know Yourself: Your Hormones

Humbling hormones

The story of a man who, due to an undiagnosed medical condition, lived without the male sex hormone testosterone for four months is shared by Dr Sarah Hill in her book *How the Pill Changes Everything: Your Brain on Birth Control*. This man said of his experience: 'Everything that I identified as being me, my ambition, my interest in things, my sense of humour, the inflection in my voice, the quality of my speech even, changed in the time that I was without a lot of that hormone.' Once testosterone was reintroduced into his body after diagnosis, he reflected on how the absence and reintroduction of small amounts of a chemical (testosterone) changed 'everything I know as myself'. He went on to say that it violated his 'understanding that who you are exists independent of any other forces in the universe. And that's humbling.'

It is indeed humbling and an important reminder that your brain creates you and that 'you' can change when your hormones change. Life makes a lot more sense when you accept that your hormones are fundamental to who you are. Hormones are critical to the health of your body and the health of your brain. Even small changes in hormone levels can have adverse effects including brain fog. As Joanne said in Chapter 1, brain fog can feel like losing yourself.

Hormonal imbalance can also lead to chronic health issues that, in turn, are associated with brain fog. Knowing how your hormones work will help you to identify how and when they influence your brain fog and your brain function. This knowledge will help you to make informed decisions to get you back to where you want to be. The good news is that making some lifestyle changes can help to get your hormones back on track, eliminating brain fog symptoms in the process. Hormones are fundamental to who you are. Anyone who has had their feelings dismissed as hormonal may bristle at that suggestion, but understanding how your hormones work will give you more control over your life, not less.

If, in addition to your brain fog, you experience any of the symptoms of hormonal imbalance discussed here then I would advise you to make an appointment with your doctor. Many hormonal issues can be detected by a blood test. As you read through this chapter, make a note of your hormonal symptoms alongside any other observations in the symptoms page at the end of this book while they are fresh in your mind. You can share this information with your doctor. This is not about self-diagnosis, it is about building up a detailed picture to help you and your doctor to decide the appropriate course of action.

Your hormones and you

Our sex and stress hormones are especially potent. It is a simple biological fact that your sex hormones have a huge influence over every aspect of 'you' – your brain, your body and your behaviour. When your hormones change, you change. Sometimes the changes are subtle and at other times the changes are quite dramatic, as Sally and her family can testify.

Sally's husband Dean describes Sally's monthly transformation. 'She became unrecognisable. She was a Jekyll and Hyde. For a few days every month we lost our funny, patient, rational Sally to this other, not very nice, sometimes downright scary person. There was no talking to her, me and the kids just had to do our best to keep out of her way. If she left the house to go shopping she ended up having a row with someone in the supermarket car park. You just couldn't speak to her; she became totally irrational.'

For Sally herself, 'It was like there had to be a blood-letting before I could feel normal again. That's probably an unfortunate turn of phrase but what I mean is I had to have a fight in order to release tension. I don't mean a physical fight but I had to rant and rave and scream, and sometimes I did throw things. I totally understand the phrase "seeing red" – I literally felt like I was inside a red haze. There was a small part of me that was looking on, that still felt like me, that would say, "What are you doing? Don't do this to yourself, stop now." But I couldn't; it was truly awful.'

Hormonal impairment does not just apply to women; well-maintained hormones are fundamental to support cognitive abilities in both men and women. While more research is needed to fully understand the exact pathways involved, we do know that hormonal changes can directly affect the ability to solve problems and the way that you navigate the physical space around you. Colette's self-described clumsiness with her stubbed toe heralding the start of her period every month comes to mind.

Despite the fact that we tend to talk about hormones in a derogatory fashion, blaming them for 'unreasonable' or 'out-of-character behaviour', our hormones are essential for survival. They play a key role in how your brain works. They are responsible for keeping your various bodily systems on the same page about what your body should be doing at any moment in time. Your hormones coordinate pretty much everything that your brain and body do, including digesting and metabolising the food that you eat, breathing, sleeping, stressing, sensing, growing and developing, as well as things we more usually associate hormones with, like your mood, ovulating, having children and sex. This means that your hormones influence your behaviour, how you think, how you perceive the world, how you feel about people and things, how you look, how you smell, how much you eat, how your immune system works and even who you find attractive.

Once you accept that biological fact, it's easier to understand how hormone fluctuations and hormonal imbalance can change you and affect how your brain works. Imbalance can occur due to illness and certain disorders. Poor lifestyle choices like smoking or leading a stressful, sedentary life with insufficient sleep will put your hormones out of whack, contribute to your brain fog and change your personality. Hormones do such a good job we only tend to notice them when they malfunction.

How do hormones work?

Hormones are communication chemicals. Your endocrine system is comprised of several glands that produce and release hormones. These chemical messengers travel, via your bloodstream, to tissues near the gland that released them and also to other further away parts of your body, where they react with target receptor sites to bring about a specific response. That feeling you get in your stomach when you feel afraid is the hormone adrenaline being released by your adrenal glands, which sit above your kidneys. Once released in response to a threat, the adrenaline travels through your blood stream to several of your vital organs including your heart, lungs and liver. On reaching its target organ, adrenaline binds to receptors to produce a specific response. Your heart will respond by beating faster and your liver cells will be prompted to break down large sugar molecules into glucose to give your muscles the boost of energy they need to fight or flee. Once adrenaline has been used for these functions it is destroyed by the liver.

Hormones are a very effective way to communicate information to multiple body systems at the same time. Just like neurotransmitters, they operate like a lock and key mechanism so that a specific hormone will only fit its target receptor. You have hormone receptors every-where in your body and in your brain, but the lock and key receptor mechanism ensures that when a particular hormone is released into the blood stream only the parts of the body that need to respond (i.e. the part with the matching receptor) will receive the instructions to carry out the intended response.

While the endocrine system is comprised of glands, it also recruits various organs that respond to, change or metabolise hormones. De-pending on the hormone released, the response could be the release of another hormone, a change in your metabolism or a behavioural response. Your metabolism influences how your body stores and uses energy from food, grows and maintains your muscles, breaks down the stored fat and how quickly you burn calories. Your hormones control all of these metabolic functions and they need to be in balance in order for you to maintain a healthy weight, which is critical for a healthy brain. Being overweight or obese increases your risk of developing type-2 diabetes, which can cause brain fog. The relationship between hormones and your behaviour works both ways. Hormone release can increase the likelihood that you will behave in a certain way and your behaviour can feed back to influence the level of hormone concentrations in your body.

The main endocrine glands that produce and release hormones are: the hypothalamus, the pituitary gland, the thyroid gland, the parathyroid gland, the pineal gland, the adrenal glands, the pancreas and the ovaries and testes. Rather than give an exhaustive description of hormonal function, the section below is a selective overview that focuses on the glands and hormones that are more likely to play a role in brain fog. I begin by talking about the first three glands on the list, which work together to form the hypothalamic-pituitary-adrenal axis (HPA-axis) because disruptions to its functioning can give rise to brain fog.

HPA-axis

The HPA-axis plays a critical role in your body's response to stress. When it is activated, cortisol is released. Chronic stress (see Chapter 8) can disrupt the healthy functioning of the HPA-axis, leading to brain fog symptoms including issues with learning and memory. Dysfunction of the HPA-axis has also been implicated in insomnia (see Chapter 7), chronic fatigue syndrome and fibromyalgia (see Chapter 5), all of which give rise to brain fog. You most probably associate cortisol with stress but this hormone is critical for life. It controls or supports various metabolic, immunological, cardiovascular and homeostatic functions. Cortisol is the most important glucocorticoid, a class of steroid hormones.

The hippocampus, which plays a critical role in learning and memory, is highly sensitive to changes in this class of steroid hormone. Dysfunction of the HPA-axis leads to high levels of cortisol. Atrophy (wasting) of the hippocampus and Alzheimer's disease are both associated with fluctuations in glucocorticoids.

Hypothalamus

Symptoms of hypothalamic conditions such as high blood pressure, insomnia and dehydration have the potential to impact on brain health and brain function.

The hypothalamus is located in the limbic brain. Its hormones control the production of many of your body's essential hormones, including those that govern sleep, stress, mood, thirst, hunger, temperature and sex drive. These hormones affect metabolism, the stress response, the immune response, reproduction, growth and lactation. The hypothalamus also controls the release of hormones from other glands including the nearby pituitary gland. For example, when a baby suckles its mother's breast, nerve signals are sent from the breast to the hypothalamus, which in turn sends a message to the front of the pituitary gland to release prolactin, which stimulates the release of breast milk.

Pituitary gland

In addition to stimulating milk production, the pituitary gland releases hormones that affect processes that play a role in brain fog, including blood pressure, metabolism, the stress response and the immune response.

Your pituitary gland is connected to your hypothalamus, which sits just above it at the base of the brain. Often referred to as the master gland, the pituitary gland can release a class of hormones called tropic hormones that affect the release of hormones from other glands. Rather than directly act on an organ, some hormones released from the front of the pituitary gland directly influence the secretion of hormones from other glands, which then go on to act on organs.

Adrenal glands

The main hormones released by your adrenal glands affect stress and immune responses (e.g. cortisol and adrenaline), blood pressure and metabolism. Adrenal hormones are often activated in situations that are physically or emotionally stressful, which means they can cloud your thinking.

Your adrenal glands, which sit just above your kidneys, have two parts which secrete different hormones. Cortisol is a hormone secreted by the outer part of the adrenal glands and adrenaline and noradrenaline are both released by the inner part. In addition to its involvement in the stress response, cortisol also controls your body's use of fats, proteins and carbohydrates, suppresses inflammation, regulates blood pressure and increases blood sugar. The main function of adrenaline together with noradrenaline is to prepare the body for fight or flight.

Pineal gland

If your pineal gland is not functioning properly it can disrupt your sleep patterns and even lead to insomnia, both of which can bring about brain fog. This is because your pineal gland, which is located next to the base of your brain, releases the hormone melatonin which effects the 24-hour biological rhythms of sleep (see Chapter 7), wakefulness and activity.

Thyroid

If your thyroid gland is not functioning well, producing either too much or too little thyroid hormones, it can lead to brain fog, anxiety or depression. Some people with an overactive thyroid gland experience brain fog symptoms including poor concentration and fatigue. While individuals with an underactive thyroid gland also experience fatigue and have difficulties concentrating, they seem to have specific issues with remembering things that they read or hear, for example the content of a conversation, radio interview or newspaper article. Your thyroid gland is butterfly-shaped and sits low on the front of your neck. Its hormones effect calorie burning, heart rate, metabolism.

Parathyroid glands

Behind your thyroid sit a group of small glands called your parathyroid glands. Parathyroid hormones constantly monitor and regulate the amount of calcium in your body.

Pancreas

Your brain relies on the production of glucose to function properly. If your blood sugar levels go out of whack the result is brain fog. Your pancreas, located behind your stomach in the upper left abdomen, produces hormones, including insulin, that help to control blood sugar levels. If your pancreas isn't working properly you will be diagnosed with type-2 diabetes which is associated with brain fog.

Type-2 diabetes

If you have type-2 diabetes, it may be the main culprit in your brain fog. Choosing to adopt a brain-healthy lifestyle will not only clear your fog but may also save your life. People with type-2 diabetes are not only at increased risk of impaired cognition, including brain fog and dementia, they are also at risk for early death. In fact, 3.4 million people around the world die every year from this preventable condition.

Type-2 diabetes is the result of a broken feedback loop which makes it difficult to control blood sugar levels because the body is unable to make enough insulin or the insulin that it makes doesn't work properly. In contrast to type-1 diabetes, type-2 diabetes is affected by your lifestyle and factors such as your age, your ethnicity and your family history. Being obese or overweight increase your risk of developing the condition. In Europe, about 60 million people are living with diabetes, which affects slightly more men than women. It is on the rise due to unhealthy diet, physical inactivity and increases in overweight and obesity – all things that we can control.

Ovaries and testes

Sex hormone levels can fluctuate for a variety of reasons and these changes can be accompanied by brain fog symptoms. The ovaries, located in the pelvis, produce female sex hormones including oestrogen and progesterone. The male sex hormone testosterone is produced mainly in the testes, located in the scrotum. While oestrogen is considered the female hormone and testosterone the male hormone, both hormones are present in both sexes. In fact, throughout the female lifetime, testosterone levels are significantly higher than oestradiol levels.

Sex hormones and brain function

Sex hormones distinguish males from females in ways that affect cognition. Before I elaborate further, it is important to remember that the fact that males and females are both human means that we are more alike than we are different.

However, the process of evolution by natural selection has of course led to other differences in men and women. The human brain contains sex hormone receptors, which means the brain and nervous system are programmed to do different things depending on which sex hormone is released. When sex hormones are released they are picked up by all of the cells that have sex hormone receptors. This means that your sex hormones simultaneously influence billions of cells in your body and your brain, affecting everything that you do and everything that makes you, you. Hormonal changes can influence what you think, feel and do.

While there is no overall difference in intelligence between the sexes, scientific research shows that each sex performs better on specific cognitive tasks. It is important not to confuse 'on average' with 'all'; when we say women on average are smaller than men it does not mean that all women are smaller than all men. That being said, on average, women are better at fluency, vocabulary, verbal memory, verbal learning, verbal cognition tasks, perceptual speed and fine motor dexterity. In essence, this means that women, on average, are better talkers, notice things quicker and are better at using their hands for fine work than men. On the other hand, men, on average, have been found to have a better visual memory and perform better at maths. Men also seem to have the edge when it comes to what psychologists describe as visuospatial abilities, which really just means moving your body or objects in the space around you. This means that men will be better, on average, at parking the car, changing lanes, remembering the colour of your neighbour's car and stuff that requires mathematical skills.

In short, while there are average differences between males and females in these specific cognitive skills, when you look at individuals, lots of males and females have the same or similar scores. You can be as good as your husband at parking the car and have super social skills, your dad could be dreadful at parallel parking but an amazing communicator and your mum could be brilliant at maths but struggle with everyday small talk.

Most of what we know about the influence of sex hormones on cognitive function comes from studies involving rats. The studies that have been carried out in humans mainly look at hormonal anomalies (i.e. when things deviate from what is expected) rather than normal hormonal function. This limits what we can say definitively.

Hormonal changes

Disturbances in cognitive function related to hormones are usually associated with women due to the fact that female sex hormones fluctuate across the ovulation cycle, during pregnancy and in perimenopause. Cognitive performance fluctuates across ovulation and across 24-hour and natural day/night rhythms. Research to date shows that both men and women are sensitive to hormonal changes. Having said that, when it comes to the impact of hormones on cognitive function, very little research in this area has been carried out on males which means it's not possible to say definitively but it is feasible that there are gender differences in terms of how hormonal changes influence cognitive function.

Oestrogen receptors are widely distributed in the brain. The hippocampus, the amygdala and the cerebral cortex all have oestrogen receptors. When sex hormones are released, they will be picked up by these receptors, influencing how they and you function. In particular, your thinking, memory, emotions and other cognitive processes will be affected.

It's a long time since I was pregnant, but I do remember experiencing what was then known as 'pregnancy brain'. I recall one incident in particular, mainly because in hindsight I realised how potentially dangerous it could have been. I was driving home from work and reached a fork-like junction which I encountered regularly. For some reason, on this particular day I was convinced that a red light and a no-entry sign meant that I had the right of way and I behaved accordingly. I not only went through a red light but also took an illegal turn. Thankfully the other cars, who were in the right, limited their response to blasting their car horns. Yet even as they did so, my first thought was the totally irrational 'What's their problem?' It took a surprising number of moments for me to realise what I had done wrong.

My behaviour on that day was most likely due to the fluctuations of oestrogen and progesterone that occur throughout pregnancy. Of course, I am not the only person ever to have experienced 'pregnancy brain' and my anecdotal experience is backed up by studies of pregnant women that demonstrate a relationship between hormonal fluctuations and the kind of deficits in attention, memory and executive function that we associate with brain fog.

In addition to sex and reproduction, female sex hormones affect your immune function, your appetite, your stress response and lots more, including your interest in new things. Oestrogen and progesterone are the main female sex hormones. Oestrogen is the hormone that we most associate with being a woman, because it affects the shape of our bodies, the growth of our breasts, our ability to reproduce, our motivation for sex and our ability to get pregnant. In contrast, progesterone promotes and coordinates nesting-related behaviours, it prepares the body for implantation and closes off the cervix to germs and sperm after conception. Broadly speaking, oestrogen is dominant during the first half of the cycle to coordinate conception and progesterone is dominant in the second half to coordinate implantation.

Oestrogen

Brain fog, memory issues, fatigue and sleep disruption are common symptoms associated with too little and with too much oestrogen. When oestrogen levels are balanced it helps to optimise the production of neurotransmitters and brain function, but problems, such as brain fog, arise when oestrogen levels are out of balance.

Oestrogens are multi-purpose messengers. There are three main types of oestrogens: oestradiol, the most important and beneficial type; oestriol, the main oestrogen produced during pregnancy; and oestrone, which is weak and produced in postmenopausal women. In addition to sex and reproduction, they affect many brain regions involved in non-reproductive functions including: cognitive function, mood, coordination of movement and pain. Fluctuations in oestrogen levels and depletion of oestrogen after natural or surgical menopause can lead to a host of changes in brain function and behaviour

Sally's 'Jekyll and Hyde' experience could be premenstrual dysphoric disorder (PMDD), which has similar but more serious symptoms to premenstrual syndrome (PMS). Causes are not fully understood but may be due to cyclical changes in hormones (i.e. reduced oestrogen before periods), fluctuations in serotonin or undiagnosed depression (PMS) or, in the case of PMDD, an abnormal response to normal hormonal fluctuations.

Sally's friend Maggi experiences pre-menstrual depression prior to her period due to too little oestrogen. Maggi's tendency to make poor decisions coming up to her period is probably also due, at least in part, to low oestrogen levels which can impair critical thinking.

Maggi's mum, who is currently going through menopause, has personally seen these cognitive symptoms worsen as she gets older and is really concerned that she is on a downward spiral towards dementia. She is not alone; brain fog is common among women going through the menopause. Not surprising really when you think of the sleep disruption and fluctuating moods on top of the gradual loss of oestrogen. Given that the fog can be quite debilitating, it is understandable that women worry that they are getting dementia. The problem is that worrying or feeling anxious or stressed about it will make the fog worse. It is important to take heart from the fact that the hormonal brain fog is temporary. Furthermore, there is no evidence that brain fog during menopause predicts dementia in later life.

As mentioned earlier, Amanda experiences clumsiness as a symptom of brain fog and points to it as one of her early signs of pregnancy. It's also a symptom that lingers for a few weeks after she gives birth. Considering that a pregnancy bump shifts a woman's centre of gravity, it makes sense that she might become clumsy in the third trimester. It's also understandable how things like her balance might be off-kilter after she gives birth, because brain signals related to posture, balance and orientation change quickly during pregnancy and after birth, challenging the brain to adjust accordingly.

But that doesn't explain Amanda's clumsiness in the first trimester. What's going on? Well, the clumsiness may be related to a rapid rise in a hormone called relaxin in the first few weeks of pregnancy. As the name suggests, relaxin relaxes muscles, joints, and ligaments during pregnancy, particularly in the pelvic region in preparation for birth.

Scientists think that a looser grip due to more relaxed wrist, hand and finger joints may explain why some pregnant women feel clumsier or more specifically why they drop objects more often than when they are not pregnant.

Progesterone

If you are a woman who has ever felt mood swings before your period, you can bet it had something to do with fluctuating hormones. When progesterone levels are high, the functioning of a chemical messenger called GABA in the brain is increased. GABA plays a role in promoting feelings of calm, good mood and sleep. Its main role is to reduce the activity of the neurons that it binds with, most probably to control the fear or anxiety experienced when neurons become overexcited. When progesterone fluctuates as it does with the ovulation/menstruation cycle, it can lead to mood swings as GABA function is affected. The mood instability experienced by many women, including myself, right before their period is likely a consequence of a drop in both progesterone and oestrogen levels. Decreased levels of progesterone that occur with menopause may be linked with low GABA function, leading to increased excitatory neurotransmitter activity which impairs sleep and results in depression and anxiety.

A balance between progesterone and oestrogen promotes sleep and feelings of calm. In contrast, when there is an imbalance of these two hormones or when progesterone drops dramatically, irritability, depression, anxiety, sleep disturbance and brain fog will ensue.

Progesterone may help protect brain cells by increasing chemicals involved in the repair of nerve cells and the formation of protective sheaths around nerve fibres as well as limiting the death of cells. Oestrogen may also protect the neurons in the hippocampus, protecting against the effects of cognitive ageing.

Testosterone

Testosterone is essential for physical and mental health and cognitive function in both men and women. Levels decline gradually with age in both sexes. Symptoms of deficiency – which include changes in cognition, memory loss, anxiety, depression and irritability – may be experienced by ageing men and women coming up to, during and after the menopause. Treatment with testosterone therapy has been shown to decrease anxiety and irritability. Unlike the menopause, which is experienced by all women, the andropause or 'male menopause' occurs only in some men and in some quarters its very existence is questioned. First described in an academic paper published in 1946 as the male climacteric, it was characterised by anxiety, irritability, fatigue, depression, memory problems, sleep disturbances, hot flushes, decreased libido and erectile dysfunction. The 'climacteric' occurs around ten years later than the menopause in women, and is associated with declines in various hormones, including testosterone. True andropause occurs only in men who have been subjected to surgical or medical castration due to advanced prostate cancer or in men who lose testicular function due to diseases or accidents.

Testosterone is known to act like an antidepressant and can also reduce anxiety. In older men, lower testosterone levels have been associated with poorer cognitive function. However, the research looking at the effect of decreased testosterone concentration on cognition is mixed. While some research links a decrease in testosterone to a decline in verbal and visual memory and visuospatial performance, the studies have been small and of short duration. More research is needed to draw strong conclusions. Nevertheless, in addition to depression, anxiety, moodiness, libido and erection issues, common symptoms associated with low testosterone levels include difficulty concentrating, fatigue and trouble sleeping. As you will learn in Chapter 6 disrupted sleep on its own is sufficient to give rise to brain fog symptoms.

The pill, HRT and anti-hormonal agents

Women taking the pill have smaller hippocampi than their counterparts who don't take the pill, according to emerging research. Shrinking of the hippocampus is linked to memory and emotional problems and is associated with Alzheimer's disease in later life. Whatever stage of life you are at, a shrinking hippocampus is not a good thing and could possibly underlie the brain fog or depressive symptoms that some women experience on the pill. While research confirms that pill-taking women have smaller hippocampi than women who don't, there is no evidence as yet linking this directly to brain fog symptoms. However, hypothesising a link is not unreasonable since the hippocampus is critical for learning and memory and any reduction in size will likely impact on those abilities. Pills using progestins derived from testosterone can have masculinising effects on women prompting unwanted hair growth and weight gain, definitely something few women would think desirable. According to research, this type of pill can also make women less fluent conversationalists but better at parking due to reduced verbal fluency and improved spatial ability.

There is scientific evidence from numerous studies which shows that women who take HRT containing oestrogen seem to have a protective effect against cognitive decline and dementia. The greatest benefit from taking HRT comes when it is started within 10 years of the menopause. Young women who experience an early menopause or premature ovarian insufficiency (POI) see the most benefit from taking HRT, as they have lower levels of oestrogen for longer. Various studies have shown that these women taking HRT have a lower future risk of developing dementia and Alzheimer's disease. Women of all ages who start taking HRT within 10 years of their menopause also have a lower future risk of heart disease, type-2 diabetes, osteoporosis and clinical depression. For the majority of women, taking HRT outweighs any risks. It is really important that all women receive individualised advice and treatment regarding their porimonopause and menopause from a doctor who is experienced in the menopause.

Research indicates that anti-hormonal agents widely used in breast cancer treatment can cause cognitive dysfunction and other changes in the brain and central nervous system. If you suspect that your brain fog might be related to this type of medication, it would be worth discussing with your prescribing doctor. Never stop prescribed medication abruptly unless instructed to do so by your prescribing doctor.

Changing hormones

In addition to changes associated with pregnancy, puberty, menstruation and menopause, the functioning of your endocrine system can be affected by other naturally occurring changes in your body influenced by your genes[12] and related to getting older. Diseases and prescription medications including opioids and steroids can affect the endocrine system too. Many people believe that herbal supplements and naturopathic medicines are harmless but both can affect endocrine organs.

St John's wort

You may have heard of St John's wort as a herbal supplement used to treat depression. People also take it for menopausal symptoms and premenstrual syndrome. Research on its effectiveness in treating depression, hormonal issues and several other conditions from ADHD to irritable bowel are mixed and inconclusive. However, research clearly shows that St John's wort interacts with various over-the-counter and prescription medications, including birth control pills, antidepressants, heart medication, some cancer medications and blood thinners in dangerous and sometimes fatal ways. My advice is not to mess with St John's wort, or any herbal supplements or naturopathic medicine without first discussing possible medication interactions with your prescribing doctor/s.

Genetics

Your genes can affect your endocrine system in a variety of ways. Extra, missing or damaged chromosomes can affect hormone production and function. The genes that you inherent from your parents can also place you at risk for diseases and conditions, some of which are associated with brain fog. For example, the risk for developing breast cancer, which is associated with brain fog, is far higher in women who inherit the BRCA1 or BRCA2 genes.

Getting older

The endocrine system actually continues to function well in most older people. However, as the years pass, most of us will accumulate medical conditions and our cells will change and may become damaged. Together, these changes may alter hormone levels and the response they trigger. Bodily rhythms associated with menstruation and ovulation also change with age. Due to age-related shrinkage, the pituitary gland doesn't function as well as it used to as we get older and this in turn can affect heart function. What's that got to do with brain fog? Quite a lot actually because your brain depends on your heart to provide the oxygen and nutrients that it needs to function well, so if this supply is compromised in any way it may affect cognition.

Diseases and conditions

Brain fog can occur if your hormones go out of balance. This can happen when the endocrine glands make too much or too little of a hormone as a consequence of some chronic diseases and conditions. If you have chronic heart, liver or kidney disease, you may experience problems breaking down hormones and this can also bring about hormone imbalance. Many of the diseases, conditions and related factors (e.g. infection, destruction caused by autoimmune diseases, medications, cancer and cancer treatments) that give rise to abnormal endocrine function are discussed in detail in Chapter 5.

Environmental factors

Keeping your hormones in balance is important for clearing brain fog. Over a thousand environmental chemicals have been identified that have the capacity to interfere with the normal functioning of your endocrine system. Endocrine disrupting compounds (EDCs) change the function of the endocrine system, affecting health adversely

EDCs work in a variety of ways that impact on the functioning of certain body systems. Some EDCs can increase or decrease hormone levels by directly interfering with how they are produced, released, stored, transported or eliminated from your body. Others can block natural hormones from working or change your body's sensitivity levels to various hormones. Some EDCs can even mimic hormones binding at receptor sites.

While more research is needed to fully understand cause and effect, the ability of EDCs to interfere with different hormones links them to numerous adverse health outcomes which are associated with brain fog or impact on brain health including: altered nervous system function, immune function and thyroid function, breast and prostate cancers, type-2 diabetes, obesity, cardiovascular problems and neurological and learning issues.

EDCs are found in air that you breathe, the soil that grows your food, the water you bathe in, drink and cook with, and the food and beverages that you eat and drink. These chemicals are also found in manufactured goods and household products. Common EDCs[13] are found in plastics and food storage materials, personal care products, toothpaste, anti-bacterial soap, children's products, textiles, clothing, old Teflon cookware, non-stick food wrappers, electronics and building materials, solvents and their byproducts and pesticides.

You can be exposed to EDCs through eating or drinking contaminated food or water. You may even be applying them directly to your skin as some cosmetics, sunscreens and anti-bacterials contain EDCs. You might have direct contact with them by touching furniture treated with flame retardant or fruit treated with pesticides. You can even be exposed to them in hospital though intravenous medical tubing.

EDCs are all around us. An exposed mother can biologically transfer EDCs to her baby through the placenta and breast milk. There is also evidence that EDCs can bring about changes in the cells that ultimately give rise to sperm and eggs. This means that the effects of EDCs can be passed on through genes from parent to child and future generations could inherit the negative consequences of exposures experienced by their ancestors, sustaining impact long after the original chemical is cleaned up or broken down.

Industrial chemicals and pesticides can make their way into the food chain by leaching into groundwater and soil and by building up in fish and animals. Traces of EDCs can build up in processed foods if they leach out of materials used in their manufacturing, processing, transportation and storage. Even the dust in your house can contain EDCs. You might be surprised to learn that naturally occurring plant compounds found in abundance in soy and soy products are classed as EDCs.

EDCs can interfere with your ability to manage stress, which is important since poorly managed chronic stress can give rise to brain fog. Most recently, researchers have turned their attention to the immune and inflammatory effects of EDCs (inflammation and its role in brain fog is discussed at length in Chapter 5). The endocrine system and the immune system often work in tandem to respond to illness. Not everyone will be affected in the same way by EDCs. Your genetic predisposition to certain health conditions as well as additional environmental risk factors will influence this. Generally speaking, chronic, high exposure poses the greatest risk in adults but infants and developing foetuses are vulnerable at lower exposures.

Hormone health

If you suspect that you have a hormonal imbalance caused by an underlying medical condition involving or impacting on your endocrine system or glands then it is important that you speak to your doctor. This is especially important if your symptoms interfere with your ability to carry out everyday activities and/or cause pain or discomfort. While hormonal imbalance can be a consequence of genetics or ageing, it is important to acknowledge that many hormonal imbalances are caused by external or lifestyle factors, which means that there are plenty of things that you can do to restore balance and clear brain fog.

The lifestyle changes covered in Chapters 7 to 10 – developing good sleep habits, managing stress, maintaining a healthy weight and healthy diet and being active – can all help to restore hormonal balance and alleviate brain fog symptoms. Even if the negative health impacts of EDCs are not fully understood or proven, it seems wise to err on the side of caution and minimise unncooooary day-to-day exposure. Avoid microwaving food in plastics, consider using glass, food-grade silicone or stainless steel to store food and drinks at home, replace old non-stick pans with newer ceramic coated ones and choose personal care products and household cleaners that are unscented.

Avoiding single use plastics is not only good for the environment, it's good for your endocrine system. The bottom of plastic bottles contain a marking to indicate which type of plastic they are made of. While plastics with recycling labels 1, 2 and 4 are considered safer because they are BPA-free,[14] it is important to remember that BPA is not the only EDC in plastics. In fact, BHPF,[15] a substance found in BPA-free plastics has been linked to similar harmful effects of BPA. It's best to avoid disposable plastic bottles altogether if you can.

Know Yourself: Your Defences

Self-defence and self-harming

Aoife has brain fog. Unlike my friend Joanne, she doesn't feel like she has lost herself to brain fog. Rather, she knows that her brain fog is a consequence of her autoimmune disease. A properly functioning immune system has the ability to distinguish 'self' from 'non-self', or, to put it another way, it can tell your body from a foreign body.

But Aoife's immune system is not functioning properly. It gets tissue or cells in her own body confused with a harmful invader that must be eliminated. It sounds like something out of a science fiction movie or the stuff of horror stories. In fact, when Ed Cohen, now a professor of women's and gender studies in Rutgers University, was first diagnosed with Crohn's disease a doctor told him, 'It's as if you're eating yourself alive.' That's a pretty scary way to explain to a thirteen-year-old boy that he has a disease where the lining of his small intestine is attacked by his own immune system, the very part of his body that is supposed to protect him.

The human immune system evolved to protect us from things in the environment, like viruses and bacteria, that can cause harm or kill us. It does a damn good job most of the time but unfortunately sometimes it gets it wrong and mistakenly attacks its own cells. This can result in autoimmune diseases, many of which are characterised by debilitating brain fog.

The first line of defence in humans is a barrier system (e.g. skin, lungs, digestive tract, tears and saliva) designed to keep infection out. If this barrier is breached your second line of defence, your immune system, kicks in. This complicated defence system does an amazing job. It doesn't just have the dexterity to defeat an incredible array of harmful invaders, it also keeps a record of every invader it ever defeated. It uses this record to recognise and destroy the invader rapidly next time it enters the body, thereby easily suppressing any future invasion by the same attackers. Unfortunately, the immune system also keeps a record when it mistakenly attacks healthy cells and continues to see them as alien, attacking them in cycles on an ongoing basis, without completely destroying the tissue.

Somewhat counterintuitively, bacteria and other microbes in your gut can support your immune system and help to protect you against infection. We also have a plethora of pharmaceuticals at our disposal which can fight infection and manage and treat disabling diseases and conditions. Unfortunately, some of these medications have side-effects that interfere with brain function and contribute to brain fog.

If you suspect that an underlying undiagnosed health condition or medication side-effects are at the root of your brain fog, make an appointmont with your doctor to discuss it sooner rather than later. As you read this chapter, use the symptom page at the back of this book to note any non-brain fog symptoms and any other relevant comments related to your suspicions. I will reiterate that keeping these notes is not about self-diagnosis; this is about building up a detailed picture to help your doctor to decide the appropriate course of action for you and with you.

What role does the immune response play in brain fog?

We are all familiar with feeling mentally under par when we have a cold, flu or other type of infection. This observation hints at a connection between cognition and the immune response to infection.

What is infection?

Infection occurs when a disease-causing organism (e.g. bacteria or virus), known as a pathogen, infiltrates your body causing harm. Depending on the infectious agent, symptoms may be non-existent, mild, moderate, severe or fatal. You'll probably know this from your personal experience of seasonal flu. Some years you may not even know you've had flu because your symptoms were mild like a cold, other years you may have been floored by fever and dreadful respiratory infection. You may know of older or more vulnerable relatives or friends who ended up with fatal pneumonia or sepsis. If your immune system's defence is successful you may remain totally unaware and have no symptoms whatsoever. If your defence system is only partially successful you may demonstrate some symptoms and then recover. However, if your immune system fails completely then you may become overwhelmed by the infection process and die.

Viruses

Once viruses enter your body they attach to a cell. Viruses contain a small piece of genetic code[16] which makes the cell replicate and so the genetic material multiplies. Viruses are very difficult to treat because they hijack the machinery in your own cells to replicate themselves.

Many viruses kill their host cell. When this happens, new viruses are released which go on to infect other cells. Recovering from a viral infection doesn't necessarily mean that the virus has gone completely. The virus may simply be dormant and reactivate years later. Cold sores, caused by the herpes simplex virus, are a prime example of a virus that can lay dormant for years only to be reactivated by sunlight, fatigue or even your period at the most inopportune moments, like your first holiday with your new boyfriend or your graduation day.

Treatments for viruses generally focus on relieving the symptoms while the immune system does its job of eliminating the infection. However, anti-viral medications are prescribed in some instances, and this needs to be early on in the infection before the virus has a chance to replicate itself. Antibiotics do not combat viral infections. Vaccines greatly reduce the risk of viral infection by working with the body's natural defences to safely develop immunity to the disease. A vaccine essentially educates the body to recognise pathogens (e.g. viruses or bacteria). Molecules from the pathogen are introduced into the body during vaccination. This allows the body to safely learn to recognise these molecules and build a supply of immune cells and antibodies that will remember how to fight the harmful invader in the future.

Some viruses change the function of the cell they've attached to and can lead to cancer by forcing the cells to replicate in an 'out-of-control' way. Cancer is a group of diseases characterised by uncontrolled cell growth. When people with cancer experience brain fog they often refer to it as cancer-induced brain fog or cancer-related brain fog. The relationship between cancer and brain fog is not yet well understood. While brain fog symptoms usually resolve when treatment ends, they can persist for some people. Everyone's experience is different and cancer-related brain fog can be caused or made worse by several factors including: stress, depression, anxiety, fatigue, poor sleep, infection, pain, anaemia, menopause and lack of proper nutrition. The good news is that most, if not all of the factors that make cancer-related brain fog worse can be addressed through life choices.

Bacteria

There are 7,500,000,000 humans and 1,000,000,000,000,000,000, 000,000,000,000 bacteria on this little planet of ours. Bacteria are literally everywhere. They are incredibly hardy organisms. They can survive in extremes of temperature and some can even survive in radioactive waste. While a few cause diseases, some deadly, most strains of bacteria are harmless to humans. Some live inside our bodies while others attack harmful bacteria and prevent us from becoming ill. Harmful bacteria can be treated with antibiotics, although overuse in recent years has led to some strains of bacteria becoming resistant. These superbugs are difficult to control and treat.

Lyme disease

Several viruses, including Epstein Barr, hepatitis C, human papillomavirus and cytomegalovirus, and bacterial infections Lyme disease and helicobacter pylori (which I have had) are associated with brain fog.

Let's take Lyme disease, which is a bacterial infection spread to humans by ticks, as an example. If caught early, most cases can be cured with a two-to-four week course of oral antibiotics. Patients whose symptoms, including brain fog, continue after treatment are said to have post-treatment Lyme disease syndrome (PTLDS).

Anita, who had PTLDS, describes her experience of brain fog. 'I did all the usual things people joke about with brain fog, like pouring orange juice on my cereal or asking my husband to get the butter out of the fire when I mean fridge. I could laugh about these blips but a lot of the time I felt like someone had poured sticky, runny toffee into my brain, letting it fill up and harden in all of the gaps and creases. It even spread into the space between my brain and my skull. At which point I would feel like I wanted to explode or crack open my skull and start chipping away at the toffee to relieve the pressure and unblock my brain.'

Brain fog occurs when Lyme pathogens, bacteria called spirochetes (they are long and coiled like a spiral spring), cross the blood brain barrier causing inflammation in the central nervous system. Symptoms include memory issues, slow processing speed, problems finding words and impaired dexterity.

Anita continues, 'Over time, as the antibiotic treatment worked, my worst symptoms abated and I could do more without getting exhausted or overloaded. I still get symptoms every so often, usually when I'm stressed, overstretched, working long hours or pushing myself too hard on the exercise front. I see that as a warning to adjust my behaviour, which thankfully reduces my brain fog symptoms.'

Any severe, systemic illness will take its toll not only on your body but also on your brain. It can often take a few months for people to get back to themselves, both physically and mentally, after a bad viral or bacterial infection. People who survive sepsis can continue to experience physical, psychological and cognitive symptoms for as long as a year after infection. It's been estimated that one in ten people who survive COVID-19 are left with lingering symptoms, including brain fog, months after infection.

If you suspect that your brain fog symptoms could be related to a viral or bacterial infection that you have or have had in the past then it is worth talking to your GP about your concerns. Researchers have identified inflammatory markers in the brains of people, like Anita, who have PTLDS.

Lyme disease is classed as an inflammatory disease. Although often discussed together, inflammation and infection are not the same thing. Infection occurs when a foreign body – in the case of Lyme disease, a bacteria – infiltrates the body, causing harm. In contrast, inflammation is your body's protective mechanism against infection or cancer.

What is inflammation?

Broadly speaking, there are two types of inflammation: acute and chronic. Acute inflammation is a short-term healthy immune response to infection or injury. It occurs in the area affected and shuts down once the injury or infection is healed. If you've ever twisted your ankle you'll recall the swelling and the pain and you might also have noticed that the injured ankle was red and hot to the touch. That is acute inflammation in action.

Acute inflammation

In very general terms, acute inflammation refers to the body's immune response to injuries, pathogens (e.g. bacteria, viruses), irritants and oxidative stress.[17] Its purpose is to eradicate the initial cause of injury to cells, clear out dead cells and damaged tissue and to start tissue repair.

Swelling, pain, redness, heat and loss of function are hallmarks of an acute inflammation. When inflammation occurs, immune cells release messengers that cause the blood vessels in the tissue to open up, allowing more blood and more immune cells to reach the injured tissue to help with the healing process. The increased blood flow is what causes the inflamed area to become red and hot. The inflammatory messengers also irritate nerve cells, causing pain signals to be sent to the brain. Pain serves a protective purpose as we naturally try to limit it, for example, by not walking on that swollen ankle.

Another sign of acute inflammation is loss of function. You know that horrible feeling when you're all bunged up with a cold and you can't smell or taste your food? That's an example of lost function. When inflammation is severe involving fever, it leads to widespread symptoms including fatigue, loss of appetite, loss of interest and cognitive dysfunction. The body is trying to make you stop and rest so that it can better fight the infection.

Chronic inflammation

Sometimes, lingering, low-grade chronic inflammation can occur. This means that the inflammation continues for a long time and is ongoing. The immune system can attack the body's own cells in the same way it would attack an invading organism. This is not healthy and can lead to inflammatory and autoimmune conditions and diseases that are often associated with brain fog.

With chronic inflammation, a shift occurs in the type of cells at the inflammation site. In addition to healing, destruction of tissue occurs. Chronic inflammation can develop anywhere in the body. Chronic inflammatory diseases such as type-2 diabetes are the most significant cause of death in the world.

Inflammation is generally associated with pain. For example, people living with the autoimmune disease rheumatoid arthritis experience pain in their joints because the immune system attacks the lining of the joints. In contrast, brain inflammation doesn't cause pain because there are no pain receptors in the brain. But don't confuse painless with harmless because inflammation can cause damage to your most vital organ. Chronic brain inflammation has been linked to depression, anxiety, Alzheimer's disease and Parkinson's disease and is associated with shrinking of the brain. Chronic brain inflammation interferes with energy production in brain cells which leads to brain fog, fatigue and memory loss. Recent research has shown that inflammation specifically alters brain activity associated with alertness, which could underlie feelings of fogginess.

Autoimmunity

While brain fog is a common complaint among people with autoimmune diseases, it can be difficult to determine the exact cause of the brain fog. This is because people with autoimmune diseases often also live with depression, anxiety and/or fatigue, all of which can also cause or contribute to brain fog. To complicate matters further, some medications prescribed to treat autoimmune disease symptoms may also exacerbate brain fog.

The autoimmune diseases most commonly associated with brain fog are: coeliac disease, autoimmune thyroiditis, multiple sclerosis, rheumatoid arthritis, Sjögren's syndrome, systemic lupus erythema-tosus (SLE) and type-1 diabetes mellitus.

Coeliac disease

Angie, who lives with brain fog, describes what life was like for her prior to receiving her diagnosis of coeliac disease two years ago when she was thirty-one: 'I felt really run down. I was so tired and found it really difficult to concentrate at work. I felt very sluggish, my thinking had become really slow and I struggled to make decisions. My tummy felt uncomfortable, bloated and crampy. My poo was really squishy and smelly. I found this really embarrassing as I work in a small office with just one toilet. I had a lot of wind and, sorry if this is too much infor-mation, but I was never quite sure whether it would be wind or actual diarrhoea. I had to make a lot of trips to the bathroom to be on the safe side. I felt really conscious about how much time I spent there.

'To be honest. I put my symptoms down to stress and feeling down because I had recently had a miscarriage. After a few months, I felt things were getting worse rather than better and my work was beginning to suffer so I paid a visit to my GP. I thought that maybe I was anaemic and might need iron tablets. After some tests I was diagnosed with coeliac disease. I had heard of it before but I thought that it just affected your gut, I had no idea that it is also associated with fatigue and brain fog.'

The most common symptoms of coeliac disease are indeed associ-ated with the gut – abdominal pain, indigestion, constipation and the unpleasant-smelling diarrhoea experienced by Angie. However, coeliac disease can also lead to more general symptoms including fatigue, weight loss and itching. Coeliac disease affects just under 1 per cent of the population in Europe and affects two to three times more women than men. A small percentage of people with coeliac disease experience neurological complications such as gluten ataxia[18] and nerve damage (peripheral neuropathy).[19] While a great deal is known about these serious, but relatively rare, neurological complications of coeliac disease, very little is known about the more common brain fog symptoms experienced by the majority of coeliac patients. Despite the fact that the cognitive impairments associated with brain fog are measurable, psychologically and neurologically valid and improve over the first twelve months when a gluten-free diet is adhered to, it is still not formally recognised.

While more research is needed, studies suggest it is unlikely that gluten directly causes the brain fog. Instead, inflammation is the more likely cause. When people with coeliac disease ingest gluten it triggers an inappropriate immune response causing inflammation, which then gives rise to the symptoms of brain fog.

Coeliac disease is associated with changes in the structure of the brain. These changes, which include small reductions in the size of brain cells and inflammation of the white matter, can result in subtle impairments to memory and attention, difficulties making decisions, as well as a general slowing – in other words, the brain fog experienced by Angie and others like her who live with coeliac disease. Like other newly diagnosed patients, Angie reported improvement in her brain fog symptoms when she began a gluten-free diet. She also found that her brain fog returned if she was accidentally exposed to gluten.

Gluten is found mainly in wheat, barley, rye and spelt and foods made from them (e.g. breads, pastas, breakfast cereals, biscuits, cakes, pies and pastries). Gluten describes a group of proteins that form sticky networks which make bread rise during baking and give that satisfying, characteristic chewy texture we all love. Essentially, the body's immune system attacks its own tissue when people affected by coeliac disease eat anything that contains gluten.

The only treatment for the disease is to adopt a gluten-free diet. If you suspect that you may have coeliac disease then speak to your doctor as soon as possible about your symptoms and ask for a test to eliminate or confirm diagnosis. If you discover you have the condition, you may find the fog lifts if you eradicate gluten from your diet completely. It's best to opt for foods that are naturally free of gluten rather than gluten-free breads, pastas etc. that have been specifically manufactured for people living with coeliac disease as they often contain a lot of saturated fats and added sugar, which means they may, in fact, be less healthy than the gluten variety. Also bear in mind that many other products that you ingest may also contain gluten, such as seasoning, sauces, dressings, tea made with tea bags, French fries, chillies, curries, envelope glue, some lipsticks, lotions, make-up products and toothpastes.

There has been a recent trend of opting for gluten-free breads and pastas as a 'healthy option' in people who do not have a coeliac diagnosis. If you have not been diagnosed with coeliac disease it is not recommended that you cut gluten from your diet. Bear in mind that the high saturated fat content in many gluten free products is, in fact, unhealthy.

Autoimmune thyroiditis

Difficulty concentrating and depression are common symptoms in auto-immune thyroiditis, which is the most common cause of an under-active thyroid (hypothyroidism). Autoimmune thyroiditis damages the thyroid through chronic inflammation, reducing its ability to produce hormones. The disease occurs more frequently in women than in men and is commonly associated with goitre and nervousness. If you've been feeling tired, sluggish, have dry skin, constipation, a hoarse voice or have had previous thyroid issues talk to your doctor about having a test.

Multiple sclerosis

Multiple sclerosis (MS) is a neurological condition where the body's immune system attacks the nervous system, destroying the white myelin sheaths that protect the brain's communication cables. Without this protective covering, the transmission of electrical signals in the brain and spinal cord are disrupted and the consequences are devastating. In addition to brain fog, symptoms of MS can include difficulties walking, vision problems, pain, bladder problems and fatigue.

Approximately 700,000 people in Europe live with MS and between 45 and 65 per cent of those will experience varying degrees of severity of what people with MS often refer to as 'cog-fog'. Problems with executive function, memory, attention, processing speed, visual perception and language are common. If you are living with MS it is important to note that only one or two domains of cognition are usually affected. Some people with MS also experience problems with controlling the expression of their emotions. MS is three times more common in women than men.

Rheumatoid arthritis

Brain fog is one of the lesser known symptoms of rheumatoid arthritis (RA), a painful autoimmune disease that causes chronic abnormal inflammation in the joints. Individuals with high levels of pain have impaired executive function. The anxiety and depression that can accompany coping with this pain may also impair cognition. When body tissue is inflamed it can send messages to the brain that produce fatigue and feelings of malaise. In a healthy immune response, cytokines – the immune system's chemical messengers – regulate how the immune system responds to threat from infection. However, inside the brain they may actually alter the activity and number of neurotransmitters, which in turn can change behaviour, emotions and energy levels. RA affects up to 1 per cent of the population and is twice as common in women as men.

Sjögren's syndrome

Problems with cognitive function are common in patients with primary Sjögren's syndrome. In fact, they are often the first clinical symptom of the disease, occurring on average two years before diagnosis. Sjögren's is a chronic systemic autoimmune disease, twenty times more common in women than men. When it is associated with another underlying auto-immune disease such as rheumatoid arthritis or systemic lupus erythematosus, it is referred to as secondary Sjögren's. Over half of all patients with Sjögren's have another autoimmune disease. If no other autoimmune disease is present then primary Sjögren's is diagnosed. Sjögren's attacks the moisture producing glands in the body. Dry eyes and dry mouth are the most common symptoms. Fatigue is a big issue in Sjögren's.

I will never forget the overwhelming fatigue that I experienced in the years preceding my diagnosis with primary Sjögren's. It was overwhelming. I felt so exhausted that keeping my eyes open was a mammoth task. The sandman quite literally set up residence in my eyes. I felt like I was forming my words in slow motion and I felt that my speech was slurred. I found it incredibly frustrating not to be able to do the things that I wanted to do. I'm a doer and being unable to do was akin to torture.

I coughed a lot at night-time and prolonged coughing fits really interfered with my sleep and my ability to function the next day. On top of this, I had agonising pain in my arms and legs. Actually, everywhere hurt. Even small movements like stirring soup on the stove felt like torture. I couldn't even put a handbag on my shoulder because the strap felt like it was burning through my skin to my bone. I stopped doing everything except my PhD. I no longer went to the gym, I stopped walking my dogs (don't worry, my husband walked them), I stopped socialising, I couldn't do any housework, even raising my arms to wash my hair in the shower had become impossibly painful. I'd gone from a high-energy, high-achieving individual who went to the gym five times a week to someone who struggled to keep her eyes open and could barely move without excruciating pain. Blood tests indicated something autoimmune was at play and an invasive lip biopsy which showed the death of salivary glands confirmed a definitive diagnosis of Sjögren's. Like many women with Sjögren's, it took several years for me to get a diagnosis and, whilst there is no cure, it is a relief to know that you are not a hypochondriac and neither are you imagining things.

Systemic lupus erythematosus

'Lupus brain fog' is the term used by people with systemic lupus erythematosus (SLE) to describe the difficulties they experience processing, learning and remembering information. Brain fog, fatigue and depression are among the most common symptoms reported by patients with SLE, a chronic autoimmune disease that causes inflammation throughout the body. SLE can involve several organs including the skin, joints and lungs. The signs and symptoms of SLE vary among individuals but a characteristic feature is a flat red 'butterfly rash' across the cheeks and the bridge of the nose. The inflammation associated with SLE can also damage the central nervous system, resulting in seizures and stroke. Globally about five million people live with SLE, which affects nine females for every one male.

Type-1 diabetes

If your blood sugar becomes unstable, swinging too high or too low, it can cause brain fog. Type-1 diabetes is an autoimmune disease characterised by abnormally high blood sugar levels. In this form of diabetes, as a consequence of autoimmune destruction of pancreatic cells, the body stops producing the hormone insulin which is essential for the production of glucose for energy and therefore a healthy brain and body. Glucose is the brain's main source of fuel, so if your blood sugar levels are off then it's easy to see how you would experience brain fog. Unlike most autoimmune diseases that disproportionally affect females, type-1 diabetes affects males and females equally – possibly because it is thought to be caused by a preceding viral infection. Type-1 diabetes represents about 8 per cent of all cases of diabetes; type-2 diabetes about 90 per cent and the remainder is made up of other types of diabetes, including gestational diabetes.

Early signs of type-1 diabetes include frequent urination, constant thirst, blurred vision, weight loss and fatigue. If you think you may have type-1 diabetes make an appointment with your doctor. If you have been diagnosed with type-1 diabetes the best way to manage your brain fog symptoms is to follow your doctor's advice about medication and diet and to be vigilant about keeping your blood sugar levels within a healthy range.

Keeping a journal of your brain fog symptoms together with a note of the food you eat and the activities that you take part in will help you to identify patterns and triggers. Some foods and activities may affect your blood sugar differently so keeping a journal could help to identify possible triggers and avoid them in the future.

What is pain and what role does it play in brain fog?

The experience of pain is commonly linked with reports of cognitive impairment, especially in individuals living with chronic, or long-term, pain. The relationship between pain and cognitive function is complex, not least because pain is often associated with stress, fatigue, anxiety and depression, which can also impair cognitive function. This makes it difficult to draw definitive conclusions about the relationship between pain and cognitive function directly. Nevertheless, understanding pain, the cognitive impairments associated with it and the possible mechanisms that underlie its impact on cognition may help us to understand and take action to minimise brain fog.

Somewhat counterintuitively, pain is integral to our defence. It serves to protect us by demanding our attention, alerting us to injury and forcing us to take protective action, usually by avoiding use of the injured part of the body or by retreating to rest the entire person.

What is pain?

I'm guessing that if I asked you tell me what pain is, you'd definitely describe it as an unpleasant physical sensation. However, if I asked you to describe your experience of a specific instance when you had significant pain, it's unlikely that you would limit your description to 'I had a sharp burning pain'. It is more likely that your description will be about how you felt and how that experience compared with past experiences of pain. Your description is more likely to run along the same lines as Dave's: 'The pain was excruciating, worse than anything I had ever experienced before. I really thought I was having a heart attack. I literally thought I was going to die, I started to panic even though I tried not to. I thought, "Is this it? Am I going to die here on my own on the side of the road?" I couldn't breathe. I barely managed to dial 999.'

Adopting this kind of approach to describing pain allows you to evaluate your current experience and make decisions about how to act. In order to consciously experience pain, your brain must receive the sensory information, form a perception of it and process the information, evaluating it both cognitively and emotionally.

Pain: sensing

The sensations of sight, sound, smell and taste occur only in special sense organs located in your head region. In contrast, your physical or bodily senses operate by detecting touch, pain, pressure, temperature and tension on your skin and internal organs. Your senses allow your body to detect changes in your external environment or inside your body. This sensory information enables your central nervous system to produce appropriate reactions and maintain the homeostasis of the systems and processes in your body that are necessary for healthy functioning. The sensation of pain differs from other sensations in that it provides information that serves a protective purpose.

Pain: nervous system

Pain is a complex sensation that is broadly categorised as inflammatory, nociceptive or neuropathic. As mentioned earlier, chemicals involved in the inflammatory response can irritate pain receptors, producing pain and inducing protective behaviours such as avoiding putting your weight on that twisted ankle. Neuropathic pain is caused by disease or injury to the nervous system itself and includes several chronic and autoimmune conditions.

Nociceptive pain, despite its unfamiliar name, is the common pain we experience when we sustain physical damage like a sports injury. You have undoubtedly experienced nociceptive pain when you've stubbed your toe, bumped your head or had a sinus infection or a bad cold. When something harms your body, information about the tissue damage is relayed from the perceived site to your brain via your nervous system.

Common pain – nociceptive pain

When something harmful comes into contact with your body, pain nerve fibres – more accurately called nociceptive nerve fibres – are activated. Information about tissue damage or potential for damage is converted to electrical signals which are transmitted via your peripheral nervous system to your spine and ultimately to your brain, where they are perceived. This information processing is called nociception. The nervous system has mechanisms for filtering the signal so activation of nociceptive nerve fibres won't always result in the experience of pain, especially if only a small number of pain fibres are activated at the same time as a large number of touch nerve fibres. Essentially, this means that there is a threshold – the nociceptors will only respond when you touch something if the stimulus is strong enough to cause injury. Nociceptive pain is acute and diminishes with healing over time.

There are two types of pain fibres, fast and slow, that can be activated during the perception of pain. You will perceive pain immediately when, for example, an injury such as a twisted ankle activates the fast nociceptive fibres which relay information to special neurons located in a particular area of your spine. You will experience a sharp stinging sensation as these fast pain fibres send a pain alerting signal that there has been or may be tissue damage.

As the strength of the stimulus increases, the slow pain nerve fibres are recruited during phase two of pain perception. They transmit information about the intensity of the pain to neurons in your spine and you will experience an aching or burning sensation. This second phase is more unpleasant than the first, is more distributed and occurs after a delay. Pain signals are sent up the spinal cord and ultimately on to various parts of your emotional brain and to regions of your thinking brain.

Chronic pain

Impaired cognitive functioning is commonly reported by individuals affected by chronic pain. Pain which persists for three to six months or longer is defined as chronic. Essentially, chronic pain means that pain signals persist even after the injury or illness that initially caused the pain has healed or gone away. Chronic pain is notoriously difficult to treat. Approximately 19 per cent of people in Europe live with chronic pain of moderate to severe intensity and only 50 per cent of these receive adequate pain management. If you live with chronic pain and feel that your pain is not being properly managed speak to your doctor and if you find that unsatisfactory, consider seeking a second opinion from another doctor or pain specialist. If you are experiencing chronic pain and have not yet seen your doctor make an appointment now.

Chronic pain can be inflammatory as in the painful autoimmune conditions described above. Chronic pain can also be idiopathic which means that there is no known cause or disease involved. Chronic pain can also be neuropathic.

Neuropathic pain is chronic by definition and can get worse over time. Several factors may contribute to neuropathic pain: abnormal activity in nociceptive nerves, sensitisation of central and peripheral nerves, impairment in mechanisms that usually filter or supress the pain response or disease activation of certain immune cells. Essentially, the system that normally regulates and controls pain malfunctions or becomes damaged, leading to neuropathic pain syndrome or chronic pain. Inherent factors (possibly genetic) may trigger neuropathic pain in some individuals.

Most conditions that cause pain have the capacity to trigger neuropathic pain in individuals who are susceptible, for example, diabetes, multiple sclerosis, shingles, HIV, cancer and vitamin deficiencies. Cancer treatment or an injury that damages nerves or nerve problems (e.g. carpel tunnel syndrome) can also trigger neuropathic pain.

Fibromyalgia

Fibromyalgia is a chronic pain condition consistently associated with brain fog. The cognitive impairments experienced by those with fibro-myalgia are commonly referred to as 'fibro-fog'. Research suggests that fibromyalgia affects how your brain processes pain signals in a way that amplifies the pain sensation. Characterised by widespread pain and musculoskeletal pain, it is often accompanied by fatigue and sleep issues such as waking up feeling unrefreshed. Fibro-fog impairs the ability to focus, pay attention and concentrate on mental tasks. People with fibromyalgia often live with additional pain, including migraine, headache, back and neck pain, stomach pain and digestive disorders including irritable bowel syndrome. Some people with fibromyalgia also experience mood or psychiatric disorders. Fibromyalgia symptoms can occur on their own or together with other autoimmune diseases including rheumatoid arthritis, SLE and Sjögren's.

My diagnosing rheumatologist attributed my pain to my Sjögren's, saying that I would have to learn to live with it. However, when I was referred to a rheumatologist at a different hospital he diagnosed me with fibromyalgia when, on examination, the lightest touch on all eighteen pressure points on my body produced excruciating pain. I learned afterwards that Sjögren's and fibromyalgia often co-occur, with some doctors believing that fibromyalgia is psychosomatic and others that it is part of rather than distinct from Sjögren's.

For a short time I debated with myself whether to mention the fibro-myalgia diagnosis or not given the controversy that surrounds it. I know that many individuals have been told that the debilitating pain that they experience is all in their head. They feel disbelieved. My view as a neuroscientist is that all pain is processed by the brain and so everyone's pain is in their head.

Whatever the diagnosis, recovery was my main goal. My rheuma-tologist advised that I exercise even though it was incredibly painful.

He also prescribed a pretty heavy-duty medication for my muscular pain and another medication for my headaches. The combination of medication and exercise worked wonders on the pain throughout my body and also improved my sleep.

Unfortunately, my headaches remained. Over time I became concerned that, while the pain throughout my body had diminished significantly, my headaches and brain fog seemed to be getting worse. My mum had dementia so I couldn't help but be concerned about my cognitive symptoms. However, I was also aware that my medication, which had a very strong sedative effect, could quite conceivably be making my brain fog worse. I made a decision to gradually taper off my medication to see if my brain fog improved. But alas, after a few weeks the pain returned with a vengeance so I resumed the medication. When I expressed my concerns to my rheumatologist he referred me to a neurologist. Thankfully there was nothing sinister on my MRI brain scan. However, the neurologist said that my headaches were not symptoms of Sjögren's or fibromyalgia. Instead he diagnosed me with chronic daily migraine.

Migraine

Migraine is a debilitating neurological condition characterised by pain, vomiting, visual disturbances and brain fog. Migraine affects 23 per cent of the population in Europe and three times as many women as men. Migraine-related brain fog usually occurs after the migraine attack but can also occur before it and can last anywhere from a few hours to several days or longer. Almost 70 per cent of people with migraine report migraine-related brain fog.

Over the last few years, together with my neurologist, through trial and error we have found a prophylactic[20] migraine treatment that works well for me. I still get headaches but they are not as severe as they once were. I exercise regularly which played a key role in allowing me to gradually come off the heavy medication that had been prescribed by my rheumatologist. Every now and again I get fibro pain with or without brain fog but I take it as a warning to pull back and do less. Usually I rest and wait it out.

Pain and cognition

There is considerable evidence that executive function, attention, memory and general cognition are affected in patients with chronic pain. With chronic pain, you may find it more difficult to control your emotions and you may also become more impulsive, responding quickly but not necessarily accurately. These kinds of deviations from your regular pattern of executive control are the kind that can really impact on relationships and make others (and you) think that you have had a personality transplant.

By its very nature, pain demands your attention. Anything else will have to compete with pain for the limited attentional resources in your brain. It may well be that pain interferes with the control mechanism in your brain that filters out things that are not relevant to the task at hand. When you have constant nerve pain it's hard to focus on anything other than the pain. But it's also hard to tune out the noise of the radio, or the car alarm so that you can pay attention to what your husband is saying. It's not surprising that people with fibromyalgia, chronic lower back pain and diabetic neuropathy report problems with attention.

Chronic pain, particularly fibromyalgia pain, seems to interfere with several types of memory (e.g. verbal, working, recall, recognition and spatial memory). Of course, the fatigue and depression commonly experienced in fibromyalgia could also contribute to or cause memory issues.

General cognition tests probe multiple areas of cognition. They are a quick method used as a first step to determine whether someone needs to be sent for further evaluation. People with chronic pain across a number of conditions are more likely to have scores that are sufficiently low to warrant further investigation.

How does pain cause brain fog?

Neural systems involved in pain and cognition are closely linked and may affect each other. Pain uses up resources and alters the brain's ability to adapt to change and the chemistry in the brain. These effects occur across a network of interconnected brain regions and may give rise to a net cognitive impairment.

Executive function depends on the frontal lobes. Animal studies show that shrinking of a specific area in the frontal lobes is associated with the onset of anxiety that is related to pain. Other studies have shown increases in the size of the amygdala that are related to pain. Essentially, the rational thinking part of your brain is reducing in size, while the fear and emotional centre of your brain is increasing in size. Research suggests that combined, these changes are responsible for pain-related cognitive impairment.

The hippocampus plays a critical role in memory and learning. Pain is a stressor and as such can suppress the growth of new neurons in the hippocampus which would have a negative effect on learning and memory. Brain-derived neurotropic factor (BDNF) is a protein which acts like a fertiliser encouraging the growth of new neurons. I like to think of it as 'Miracle-Gro' for the brain. Pain seems to bring about a reduction in the amount of fertiliser circulating in the brain, resulting in an environment less conducive to growing new neurons and new brain connections between neurons.

Pain processing and cognition share several of the same neurotransmitter systems. It is possible that brain fog is a consequence of pain-related changes in chemical messengers and the transmission of signals. Brain fog experienced with chronic pain could also simply be a consequence of competition for limited resources.

Pharmaceutical arsenal

Pharmaceuticals can be deployed in the fight against and treatment of infection, pain, autoimmune disease, cancer and other health issues. Unfortunately, some treatments can backfire in the sense that they can have side-effects that give rise to or exacerbate brain fog symptoms. Symptoms that, for some, are almost harder to live with than their original symptoms.

Chemotherapy

Various types of chemotherapy medications are used to kill cancer cells and stop them reproducing and spreading in the body. During and after treatment, about 70 per cent of patients experience brain fog, the most common side effect of chemotherapy usually referred to as 'chemo brain' or 'chemo fog'. Thankfully, the symptoms usually resolve several months after treatment ends. Unfortunately, however, for one in every four originally affected, the symptoms can persist for years, in some cases up to fifteen years. Executive function, attention, working memory and processing speed are the most common cognitive domains affected by chemotherapy. Women receiving treatment for breast cancer are particularly vulnerable. Some breast cancer patients report brain fog prior to chemotherapy, which could be caused by the tumour, stress or surgical interventions. Even when this is the case, chemotherapy is associated with further decline in cognitive function over time.

Chemotherapy can reduce the size of the brain and bring about changes in activity patterns. Scientific research to date suggests that the brain fog associated with chemotherapy occurs as a consequence of brain inflammation and a reduction in the growth of new neurons in the hippocampus. The memory and attention problems that patients experience are most probably a consequence of damage to the hippocampus and the frontal lobes.

While chemotherapy is designed to kill rapidly reproducing cancer cells, it can also kill healthy cells. Chemotherapy medications used to treat breast, ovarian, colon and rectal cancer are also toxic to several types of brain cells. Some chemotherapy medications can disrupt neural communication by causing damage to the myelin sheaths that cover the communication cables (axons) between brain cells, which will interfere with the transmission of signals.

Other medications

Unfortunately, medications prescribed to treat pain, autoimmune diseases, anxiety and depression can have brain fog as a side-effect or make existing brain fog symptoms worse. Other medications associated with brain fog include antihistamines, blood pressure medications, anti-nausea tablets and some sleeping tablets. In addition, drug interactions from taking multiple medications prescribed for a variety of conditions can cause brain fog.

Not all of these medications will impair cognitive function but if you feel that your brain fog may be a side-effect of your medication speak to your prescribing doctor; there may well be other options to explore. Never stop taking prescribed medication without consulting with your doctor. Suddenly stopping some medications can have catastrophic health implications and could even cause death. For example, abruptly discontinuing certain heart medications can actually cause a heart attack.

Ancient allies

Trillions of microbes live inside you. If I'm honest, this is not something I like to think about. I have a very visual imagination. I really don't like looking at images of microbes under a microscope. It gives me the same creepy feeling that looking at a fossil or microscopic images of bed bugs give me. I am literally getting the creeps as I type this but I really must continue because some of the microbes in your gut defend you against pathogens and may play a role in your brain fog. They certainly play a role in anxiety and depression which are associated with brain fog.

Microbes are literally everywhere. They are masters of reproduction and think nothing of interbreeding and genetic reinvention. They are capable of mutating every twenty minutes. Millions of years ago, bacteria and animals, including humans, became allies. We formed an alliance towards a shared cause, our mutual survival. Our warm, moist gut with its endless supply of rations became the perfect billet for beneficial bacteria. In return for food and lodgings, these bacteria help digest food and defend us against pathogens in what could be described as the earliest form of defence in germ warfare.

These beneficial bacteria don't just fight off rogue microbes, they make the most out of every last calorie that we ingest and even produce some of the vitamins that we need. When taken together, the battalions of microbes living within your gut are called microbiota. In addition to bacteria, there are battalions of viruses, single-celled protozoans, ancient life-forms called archaea and yeasts. In fact, Anderson, Scott and Cryan, authors of *The Psychobiotic Revolution*, argue that we are actually hybrid creatures: part human, part microbiota, with microbial genes outnumbering our human genes 100 to 1. It kind of gives me the shivers to think about it but this seething microbiota is like another organ in your body.

Gut-brain-axis

The gut-brain-axis (GBA) operates in two directions, linking the central nervous system (CNS) and the enteric nervous system (ENS), which consists of a net-like system of neurons that control the function of the gastrointestinal (GI) tract. The microbes in your gut use your nervous system, your endocrine system, your immune system, your circulatory system and your lymphatic system to speak to your thinking and emotional brains. Your GI tract operates on autopilot without the need for conscious engagement of your thinking brain. All of the systems interact with each other so talking about them in isolation is a little artificial.

Your microbiota communicate directly with the nerves surrounding your gut, which, as I mentioned earlier, is sometimes referred to as your second brain. Research suggests that gut microbiota play a role in regulating anxiety, mood, cognition and pain. So paying heed to and modulating your gut microbiota may help to minimise brain fog by minimising anxiety and depression which are commonly associated with it.

When you respond to cravings, you may well be answering the call of the microbes in your gut. Microbes create cravings in one of two ways. They can use the stick approach by producing toxins that make us feel bad if we don't ingest what the microbes need. They can also use the carrot approach by changing our taste buds, stimulating opioid and endocannabinoid receptors[21] and releasing feel-good hormones (e.g. dopamine and serotonin). Microbial cravings can make us miserable or happy depending on which technique is employed. The hormonal shifts that occur during pregnancy also change the microbiota in the expectant mother's gut which bring about the crazy cravings that have long been associated with pregnancy. Responding to cravings isn't always in our best interest, as those who have developed chronic health conditions as a consequence of life-long cravings for chocolate, cakes and fatty foods can attest.

Gastric bypass surgery is a radical way to lose weight. It is considered the 'gold-standard' in surgical weight loss by many. Don't worry, I'm not going to suggest that you have your stomach partitioned so that you can feel full after eating less. But surprisingly it can tell us a lot about microbial cravings. Most of our knowledge of how microbes manipulate us through cravings comes from research with mice, who are easier to study than humans, and flies who only have a few different bacterial species. I should warn you at this point that I'm about to delve into the 'creepy' realm again with a cat and mouse story. If you can stick with me and put your disgust on hold I'm sure you'll be as fascinated as I am by the power of microbiota.

To say that cat pee has an unpleasant odour is putting it mildly. Mice find it repulsive too and generally scurry away from it, which is a good job because it contains a parasite called toxoplasma which can bring about a mouse's demise. How does that happen and what has it got to do with microbial cravings? Well, mice that have become infected with the parasite actually come to crave cat pee which means they will most likely become cat lunch. What's devastating for the mouse is nourishing for the cat and essential to the lifecycle of the toxoplasma. Makes you thankful that you crave the less imminently life-threatening Dairy Milk and Krispy Kremes. While they may taste nicer than cat pee, giving into your cravings for sugar and saturated fats may also contribute to your demise; it will just take longer than cat pee.

Gastric bypass surgery brings about a major shift in gut microbiota. This shift is accompanied by, you've guessed it, a major shift in food cravings. After surgery, people stop craving sweet and fatty foods. The success of this method in terms of weight loss is most probably not due to the reduced stomach size but more likely due to altered cravings. That knowledge is just as humbling to me as the man who lived without testosterone's discovery that small amounts of a hormone could have such a drastic influence on his personality and his sense of self. Thankfully you don't have to live at the mercy of your microbial cravings, I'll share some simple ways to build a healthier microbiota in Chapter 10.

When your microbiota encounter a pathogen it alerts your immune system and launches an attack. It will try to starve or poison the dangerous intruder. At this point, your second brain has been put on high alert and steps into action to purge your system of the pathogen, telling you to find a bathroom quickly while you are filled with feelings of anxiety. Your immune system, together with your microbiota, can protect you against pathogens never encountered before. How brilliant is that?

We are hard-wired to engage in 'illness behaviours' that encourage us to withdraw to our beds to rest and reserve energy to fight whatever bug has breached the microbiota defences. If this type of withdrawal behaviour endures for extended periods it is akin to, or even becomes, depression. Depending on the levels of inflammation, you might alternate between anxiety and depression, both of which are associated with brain fog. Of course, external events and experiences can lead to depression and anxiety and they in turn can bring about negative changes in your gut microbiota, which can channel anxiety and depression back into your brain.

Single-celled bacteria can form great military bases in the gut, comprised of several different species that can live together harmoniously in a biofilm[22] while also aiding your immune response, protecting you against pathogens. The various species communicate with each other using molecules including neurotransmitters. They work so well together they act like a multicellular organ. A well-established compatible biofilm can defend you against pathogens, leaving your gut inflammation-free for a lifetime. However, if your microbiota become unbalanced this can lead to inflammation, cognitive decline, depression and anxiety.

While on the one hand, gut bacteria can protect us against pathogens, on the other they can also give rise to low levels of inflammation and anxiety. The immune system uses cytokines to signal the alarm and coordinate the response of other immune cells. Some cytokines are inflammatory and others are anti-inflammatory. If inflammation becomes chronic, over time depression and anxiety can set in. Stress can also impair the effectiveness of your immune system. During the stress response, in an effort to conserve energy your brain dampens down the immune response. This means that pathogens can sneak in, causing infection or causing your gut to leak. A healthy gut forms a barrier that tightly controls what gets into the bloodstream (e.g. nutrients). An unhealthy gut may become more permeable allowing partially digested food, toxins and pathogens through to the bloodstream, which, in turn, can cause further inflammation. The sicker you get, the sicker you will get, and the more likely you will become depressed.

The nerve fibres throughout your digestive tract can communicate with the hypothalamus in your brain. In Chapter 4 I introduced the hypothalamus as a key gland in your endocrine system. Located in your emotional brain, the hypothalamus bridges the endocrine and nervous systems. It can breach the blood brain barrier using special nerve cells to sample blood for signs of inflammation. Immune cells in your gut tag both beneficial and pathogenic microbes by snipping off bits which are carried through your circulatory and lymphatic systems. Your hypothalamus responds to all tags but has a prolonged and strong response to potentially dangerous pathogenic tags and sends alarm signals to your pituitary and adrenal glands. This HPA-axis (hypothalamus-pituitary-adrenal) is one of the key ways that your gut communicates with your brain. The HPA-axis releases cortisol and other stress hormones in response to the inflammatory markers. Chapter 8 explores the stress response and its relationship with brain fog, anxiety and mood in considerable detail.

So there you have it, the immune system, inflammation, pain, gut microbes and pharmaceuticals do an amazing job of defending us against infection. However, autoimmune responses, prolonged pain, ongoing inflammation, disrupted microbiota and medication side-effects can bring about brain fog indirectly through anxiety and depression or by suppressing the growth of new neurons and connections between them.

Part Two
Power

The best way to win is
not to fight at all.

The Art of War – Sun Tzu

6

Power:
Brain Health

Brain health

I'm guessing that you brushed your teeth this morning. I'd also stake money on your intention to brush them again this evening. Now answer this question honestly: did you consciously, *consciously*, do something for your brain health today? Anything? Chances are that the health of your brain doesn't figure in your daily routine. That's kind of crazy when you think about it.

Of course, dental health is super important because you need your teeth to eat, to speak and to smile. But you need your brain for *everything*. There isn't one thing that you can do without your brain. You can't stand, sit, talk, walk, shop online, post on Instagram, laugh, cry, love or lie without your brain. Come to think of it, you can't even brush your teeth without your brain. Brain health matters.

As a child, you may have learned about a complex concept called investment. And even if you didn't, you will have engaged in it from a young age. Investment means time spent now engaging in a particular activity, like brushing your teeth, reaps future benefits – in this case, healthy teeth for longer. You will also have learned that if you engage in additional activities such as flossing, regular visits to your dentist and avoiding sugary drinks that you will minimise your risk of toothache and tooth decay. As an adult, you realise that even if you fastidiously follow your dentist's advice, it doesn't come with an absolute guarantee and you may have pain or need dental work but you know that you will be in a far better position as you go through life than you would have been without a daily dental health habit.

The same applies to brain health. We now know that there are things that you can do each and every day that boost the health of your brain. Just like dental health, adopting a daily brain health habit doesn't come with an absolute guarantee but we do know that your brain will be in better shape than it would be otherwise.

Your brain fog symptoms occur because your brain is challenged by one or more of the following: poor sleep, chronic stress, poor diet or nutritional deficiencies, underlying medical condition/s, fluctuating hormones, medication or other factors known to give rise to brain fog. The good news is that your brain has the capacity for resilience in the face of challenge provided you give it a helping hand by adopting a brain-healthy lifestyle. By harnessing the power of brain health, you may negate the need to fight the fog. A healthy brain can maintain its performance even in the face of considerable challenge.

Harnessing your brain's natural capacity for resilience can optimise your everyday brain performance, protect your cognitive functions and minimise brain fog symptoms. Your brain also has an amazing ability to adapt and change across your lifespan. This flexibility, called neuroplasticity, allows you to learn new things, adapt to changes and challenges in your life and your environment and even compensate for brain diseases and brain injury.

Resilience

Your brain is constantly changing. Your behaviours, your experiences and the life choices that you make each and every day continue to shape it at any age. What you do and, just as importantly, what you don't do influence how resilient your brain can be in the face of challenges, including many of those that give rise to brain fog. I like to think of adopting a brain-healthy life as investing in brain capital that not only optimises your performance in the here and now but also builds reserves that can be cashed in to cope with or compensate for future disease, damage or decline.

The idea that the brain can be resilient in the face of challenges such as disease, ageing and even injury stems from the repeated observation that the same brain injury or the same amount of brain disease can result in different symptoms or outcomes. For example, a head injury of the same magnitude can result in completely different levels of cognitive impairment and different recovery trajectories in different patients. Some people also seem to be able to tolerate more age-related brain changes and even disease-related pathology (e.g. Alzheimer's disease or multiple sclerosis) than others while still maintaining cognitive function. Scientists, including myself, who carry out research in this area use the concept of reserve to account for this resilience.

In an economic recession, savings can get you through a tough patch. In nature, animals that hibernate stock up on stored energy that they can draw on over winter. Our brains can also have reserves, which can be drawn upon in the face of disease, damage, ageing and other factors that challenge the brain. To explain this phenomenon, scientists draw a somewhat artificial but useful distinction between brain reserve and cognitive reserve. One way of thinking about this distinction is that the brain reserve is the hardware and the cognitive reserve is the software. Brain reserve describes the physical stuff (i.e. grey matter and white matter) and cognitive reserve describes the brain's ability to use this physical stuff to continue to function properly and get things done when challenged by improvising or finding alternative, more effective or more efficient ways of working.

You could also think of brain reserve as the car and cognitive reserve as the amount of oomph or power the car has to accelerate quickly and handle sharp corners. Some cars have enough power in reserve to make a sudden acceleration, but it's also possible to soup up a car engine to give it extra power so that it has enough in reserve to make that acceleration.

The same applies to brains. Not all brains have the power to do what you need to do so you can't perform at the level required to cope with the challenge of being sleep deprived or overstressed, for example. Depending on the nature and severity of the challenge, this can result in cognitive impairment. The good news is that there are ways that you can soup up your brain to give it the power, the resilience, the cognitive reserve to cope with challenges without experiencing brain fog.

The brain has an inbuilt, but limited, capacity to retain brain function in the face of a challenge. This is called 'neurological reserve' and it allows the brain to reorganise itself to compensate for brain atrophy and loss of brain cells and connections. The brain does this by rerouting communication pathways to avoid damaged areas. It can also adapt undamaged areas to take on functions that were once carried out by the area now damaged by disease. Our lifetime experiences can replenish reserves. This typically means that people who build reserves through brain-healthy life choices can minimise the impact of medical conditions and other challenges on their cognitive function for longer.

Let's take multiple sclerosis as an example of a challenge to the brain. Unfortunately, this inbuilt capacity can't keep pace with multiple sclerosis disease activity and when neurological reserve is exhausted symptoms such as fatigue, numbness, muscle spasms and brain fog appear. But this is where brain reserves and cognitive reserves built up through brain-healthy lifestyle choices come in. Here's why. All other things being equal, people with multiple sclerosis who have high cognitive reserve lose less cognitive function – or, to put it another way, have less severe brain fog – than those with less cognitive reserve for the same amount of brain lesions and atrophy. Brain-healthy life choices and experiences can increase cognitive reserve and boost brain reserve. This gives you better odds of beating brain fog if life throws you a curve ball in the shape of one of the many medical conditions associated with cognitive dysfunction. Maximising your brain health is like giving your neurological reserve a new lease of life.

Brain reserve

Brain reserve is the structural stuff: grey matter, white matter and the thickness of the cortex. Brain reserve refers to the actual differences in the physical brains of two people that might explain how one individual has greater tolerance than another to brain injury or brain volume loss caused by ageing or disease.

The overall volume of the human brain shrinks as we age, beginning anywhere from our mid-thirties to our mid-forties. From then onwards, we all lose a little brain volume each year through a process called 'atrophy'; hit sixty and the rate of that atrophy accelerates. Brain atrophy describes the loss of brain cells and the connections between them. Your brain can atrophy by about 2 per cent every ten years, leading to less brain and a loss of function. In addition to dealing with the challenge/s causing your brain fog, your brain also has to cope with the effects of age-related atrophy which can happen in just one part of the brain or can occur across the entire brain, leading to a variety of symptoms and functional loss depending on the area or areas affected.

Let's take Alzheimer's disease, for example. Not everyone with Alzheimer's disease will have the same level of cognitive impairment; when you compare people with a diagnosis of Alzheimer's and with different levels of cognitive impairment, you find that these differences are related to the size of the individual's brain rather than to the amount of disease within it. It is not the amount of disease in the brain that accounts for differences in cognitive impairment, it is the amount of intact brain.

To put it simply: brain size matters. Of course, it is important to point out that Alzheimer's disease is a progressive neurodegenerative disease. As the disease progresses, the amount of diseased brain will increase and the amount of intact brain will decrease until a certain point is reached where the intact brain can no longer maintain normal cognitive functioning and dementia symptoms will appear. But an individual with high reserve will hold on to cognitive functions for longer than an individual with low reserve.

Brain reserve means that the brain's structural characteristics provide resilience against the wasting associated with the disease. The greater your brain volume, the more neurons and connections that you have, the longer you can resist the impact of damage or disease on your functioning.

Brain maintenance

The latest thinking is that it is possible to maintain your brain reserves (i.e. stop it shrinking or at least slow it down). Your brain will still atrophy as you age but you can counteract this wasting by engaging in brain-healthy activities that promote the brain's ability to adapt, reorganise itself and grow new neurons and new connections between brain cells. Of course, your brain will function best if it is free of disease but the good news is that various lifestyle factors can help you to resist the effect that disease can have on your brain function and to avoid or ameliorate brain fog.

Brain maintenance contributes to your current levels of brain reserves. Certain activities such as physical exercise and engaging in activities that stimulate the brain, like learning a language, an instrument or a dance routine, are actually linked with changes in the brain itself. Increased cognitive activity may help to preserve the volume of your whole brain and particularly the size of the hippocampus, the part of your brain involved in memory and learning. Some people maintain their brains (and brain reserves) more successfully than others and this phenomenon may be down to differences in their life experiences.

Cognitive reserve

Cognitive reserve refers to the plasticity or flexibility of cognitive networks in the face of disruption caused by ageing, injury, disease or other challenges including those that bring about brain fog. It is concerned with how the brain functions rather than the structural brain size. Let's consider Sarah and Nadia, who are both 75 and have the same amount of brain reserve. Sarah can tolerate more age related brain changes than Nadia because she engaged in activities that 'souped up' her brain; in other words, Sarah has more cognitive reserve than Nadia which allows Sarah's brain to cope with or adapt to the disruptions.

Brain atrophy and reserve are linked to many modifiable factors. Adopting a brain-healthy approach to life that excludes smoking and includes regular physical exercise, social engagement and mental stimulation, together with a healthy diet and optimal amounts of sleep and stress, may help you to beat brain fog by boosting reserves and preventing or slowing down the rate at which your brain shrinks.

Neuroplasticity

Your brain is unique, crafted by the experiences that you offer it and the demands that you place on it each and every day. Your brain is a dynamic organ that not only influences your behaviour but is also influenced by your behaviour.

Your brain is incredibly adaptable. It can change and reorganise itself by growing new connections between brain cells. This flexibility, called neuroplasticity, is a fundamental feature of the human brain. It's not exclusive to humans but the human brain does appear to excel at adaptation. While genetics determine overall brain size in humans and chimpanzees, the human brain is more responsive to environmental influences than the chimpanzee brain, allowing it and its behaviour to constantly adapt to changes. We afford a lot of importance to genes, but lifestyle and life experiences are critical to determining the shape of the brain, how it grows and how it performs.

Neuroplasticity is the brain's capacity to change with learning and in response to novelty, challenge and injury. It occurs in response to injury to compensate for lost function and to maximise existing function. The brain can actually repair itself naturally. It does this by sprouting new projections on communication cables in order to re-establish lost connections or form new ones. The brain can also co-opt undamaged areas to take over functions of damaged areas and it can even generate new neurons. Neuroplasticity occurs at the beginning of life when the immature brain organises itself and in adulthood any time something new is learned or memorised. The take-home message is that you can change your brain through experience. Learning can shape it, rather like exercising can shape your muscles.

We hear a lot about physical health and mental health, which is fantastic and has had a huge impact on people's quality of life. But brain health rarely features in public or private conversation and I want to change that because adopting a brain-healthy life could change millions of lives for the better and has the potential to eradicate or vastly reduce the impact of brain fog. Physical health, mental health and brain health are interlinked and influence each other but, given that your brain is essentially your master controller, prioritising brain health means your physical and your mental health will benefit. Adopting a brain-healthy life is not about being brainy, rather it is about being smart enough to look after your most precious gift so that it can do its job of looking after you.

In Chapter 1, Joanne described her experience of brain fog as losing herself. This is really not surprising because your brain is fundamental to who you are. Your brain supports you in the things that you do each day that define you. It really is quite astonishing that nearly all of us have excluded our most important and most complex organ from our healthcare routine. You can harness neuroplasticity and build reserves to bid farewell to brain fog and find yourself again, or, if you so desire, you can fashion a new and improved you that thinks sharper, faster, better.

The good news is that you are probably already doing things every day that benefit your brain and build resilience. It's also likely that there is so much more that you can do. You need to consciously incorporate brain-healthy habits into your daily routine to boost reserves that your brain can draw on in the face of challenges. There are also things that you need to stop doing to keep your brain healthy. Reading this chapter has expanded your knowledge of brain health. Part Three will build on this knowledge, giving you lots of practical tips for living a brain-healthy life.

Part Three
Change

Change represents opportunity.

The Art of War – Sun Tzu

7

Change: Sleep

How good is your sleep?

Are you sleep deprived? If you are, then there is a very real chance that loss of sleep or poor sleep quality is the cause of, or, at the very least, contributing to your brain fog. If sleep loss is the main driver of your brain fog you could eliminate your symptoms by prioritising sleep. The longer you have had sleep problems, the longer it will take to make up for the loss and restore focus and clarity to your thinking.

Sleep loss, irrespective of its cause, doesn't just make you sleepy during the day. It can make you forgetful and interfere with your ability to concentrate, pay attention and learn new concepts. Ongoing sleep loss can also make you feel clumsy, irritable, moody, demotivated, depressed and leave you with food cravings and a bigger appetite than usual but no desire for sex. Yet many of us, myself included, voluntarily deprive ourselves of sleep just to binge-watch a show or surf social media. According to the World Health Organization, we are in the midst of a sleep-loss epidemic with one in three people not getting enough sleep.

Thankfully we don't need to wait for a vaccine for this epidemic. If you are sleep deprived, you have the power to change your behaviour to ensure that you get enough good quality sleep each night to restore your brain function to optimum levels and support brain activity each day. This chapter gives you the basics on how sleep works and how it affects your brain function. The assessments will help you to identify factors that may be interfering with your sleep. There are also lots of practical tips to improve your sleep habits in order to reduce your brain fog symptoms.

Assessment: Your Sleep Profile

- How many hours sleep do you get on average each night? _____
- Do you regularly take a nap? Yes __ No __
- If yes, how many minutes do you usually nap? _____
  At what time? _____
- How many hours sleep do you get in total on average in each 24 hour period? _____

The amount of sleep we need changes across our lifespan[23] and it also varies between individuals. A good rule of thumb is seven to nine hours for adults aged eighteen to sixty-four years and between seven and eight hours for adults over sixty-five. Everyone is different, so these are just guidelines. Some people will need more and some less but it is not recommended to have fewer than six hours if you are aged between eighteen and sixty-four years, or fewer than five hours if you are aged over sixty-five. Too much sleep is not recommended either, so no more than eleven hours for eighteen to twenty-five-year-olds; no more than ten hours for twenty-six to sixty-four-year-olds and no more than nine hours for those over sixty-five. These recommendations are for each twenty-four-hour period and can be taken in one long night-time sleep or can be split between night-time and a daytime nap. Some people will thrive on sleep in one single block at night-time, whereas others are at their best when they sleep for 6.5 hours at night and nap for 90 minutes during the day.

Your sleep is likely of good quality if you:

- Fall asleep within thirty minutes of going to bed.
- Spend no more than 15 per cent of your time in bed awake.
- Wake up no more than once per night and fall back to sleep within twenty minutes.

How you feel when you wake and throughout the day is also a good indicator of whether you are getting sufficient good quality sleep. Brain fog symptoms aside, do you wake up feeling refreshed and revitalised, ready to start the day, or do you feel sluggish and sleepy? Do you depend on coffee to get you through the day? Do you find yourself nodding off while driving or reading? Are you accident-prone? Do you feel irritable? If you answer yes to any of these questions, it is likely that you are getting insufficient sleep or your sleep is disrupted or of poor quality. Keeping a log of your sleep is a great way to get to know your sleep patterns and gain insight into whether poor sleep is contributing to, or the main cause of, your brain fog.

Complete in the morning	Day 1	Day 2	
Day (Mon, Tues, etc.)			
1. I went to bed last night at (time)			
2. I woke this morning at (time)			
3. I got out of bed at (time)			
4. I felt a) refreshed; b) somewhat refreshed; c) tired; d) groggy			
5. I had # hours, # minutes sleep, e.g. 06h 35m			
6. Last night I fell asleep after # minutes a) easily; b) with difficulty			
7. In the hour before bed I (list what you did, e.g. watched TV, took a bath, read a book, checked social media, online, worked, etc.)			
8. I woke during the night # times for # minutes			
9. I was woken by (list internal and external factors, such as a dream, thoughts, need to urinate, pain, dog, noise, too hot, too cold, breathing issues, coughing/snoring, etc.)			

Assessment: Sleep Log

Keep a sleep log for one week to help you to identify any patterns or personal habits that help or hinder your sleep quality. If you have a wrist activity tracker or sleep app on your phone or on your watch use it to help you to complete this chart. It will be really helpful to have this information before you begin the 30-day plan.

	Day 3	Day 4	Day 5	Day 6	Day 7

Complete in the evening	Day 1	Day 2	
10. I exercised for # minutes today			
11. I exercised at (time)			
12. I consumed # caffeinated drinks			
13. I consumed caffeinated drinks at (time/s)			
14. I consumed # units of alcohol			
15. I napped for # minutes at (time)			
16. I felt: a) alert; b) tired; c) drowsy Answer for morning, afternoon and evening	M: A: E:	M: A: E:	
17. My mood was: awful (0) to great (5)			
18. Throughout the day I . . . (Answer yes/no)			
a) had trouble concentrating			
b) had difficulty shutting out distractions			
c) had trouble sustaining attention			
d) had trouble recalling information			
e) had trouble taking in new information			
f) felt irritable			
19. I took these medications			
20. I had my evening meal at (time)			
21. I consumed my last caffeinated drink at (time)			
22. I consumed my last alcoholic drink at (time)			

Sleep Log reproduced from 100 Days to a Younger Brain *(2019) with permission from Orion Spring*

Assessment: Sleep Disruption

At the end of the week, use the table that follows to list each factor from question nine of your sleep log on a separate line under the column 'I had trouble sleeping because . . .'. Then record the frequency with

Day 3	Day 4	Day 5	Day 6	Day 7
M: A: E:	M: A: E:	M: A: E:	M: A: E:	M: A: E:

which each factor disrupted your sleep. If you did not experience a disruption this week, check the 'not this week' column. However, if you feel that you did experience disruption 'in the last month' then check that box instead and score as follows:

- Not during the past week = 0
- 1 or 2 times during the past week = 2
- 3 or more times during the past week = 3
- Less than once a week over the past month = 1

Sleep Disruptions	Based on your Sleep Log this week			In the past month	
I had trouble sleeping because:	Not this week	1 or 2 times	3 or more times	Less than once per week	Score
Total Score					

Total score = _____

What your score means

If total score is:

- 0 = no sleep disruption
- 1 to 9 inclusive = low sleep disruption
- 10 to 18 inclusive = moderate sleep disruption
- greater than 18 = high sleep disruption

The rhythm of life

The human brain evolved in a world of cyclical patterns and rhythms determined by the configuration of the earth with the solar system. Tides are driven by the moon's monthly orbit of the earth and the annual revolution of the earth around the sun is the source of seasonal fluctuations in temperature and rainfall. One complete rotation of the earth on its axis takes twenty-four hours, giving us the alternating pattern of day and night. The human brain has adapted to this cyclical environment in many ways, the most obvious being our twenty-four-hour sleep–wake cycle.

Cycles of various durations are found throughout the nervous system and in almost every tissue in the human body. The period of time it takes to go through the characteristic peak and trough of a single cycle varies enormously. Just like the sleep–wake cycle, body temperature and some hormone secretions follow a circadian rhythm, which means the time interval separating one peak or trough from the next in their repeating cycle is about twenty-four hours. Bodily rhythms, such as respiration and brain wave oscillations that have a period of less than twenty-four hours between peak and trough, are referred to as ultradian rhythms. Rhythms that cycle over more than twenty-four hours such as the ovulatory/menstrual cycle are referred to as infradian rhythms. The timing of these rhythms affects numerous critical functions including metabolism and immunity.

You will function best when your natural rhythms flow without disruption. This means it is best to work with, rather than against, your body clocks. Yes, you have multiple body clocks throughout your body and brain. Each of these innate timing devices have their own timetables but they also work together in an organised way. A central pacemaker, about the size of the tip of a pen but comprised of tens of thousands of brain cells, is located in your hypothalamus. I like to think of this pacemaker, which is called the suprachiasmatic nucleus (SCN), as a conductor ensuring that each clock keeps its own time in a way that creates the sweet music of life. It sends signals along outgoing pathways to various tissues, glands and parts of the brain to regulate the cycles of a multitude of physiological and behavioural functions, such as ovulation, hunger, temperature and the phases of sleep.

All of your body clocks are made of proteins that interact in cells. Specific genes are responsible for making the clock components. These genes interact with each other in a complex way, generating rhythmic fluctuations of gene expression. The 'clock genes' act like cogwheels in a mechanical clock. Activation of the genes involved occurs in a positive–negative cycle (e.g. sleepiness–alertness) with the activation of each gene regulated by the last one in the sequence. In the case of circadian rhythms, one cycle takes twenty-four hours.

Rhythms of the night

The timing of sleep is mainly controlled by this internal body clock that cycles between sleepiness and alertness, making you feel either drowsy or energised. For most people, the greatest dip in alertness occurs between 2 a.m. and 4 a.m. when most of us are asleep. Another dip occurs after lunch between 1 p.m. and 3 p.m. when many of us crave a nap. While this clock operates independently of how much sleep you've had or how long you have been awake in the preceding period, you will notice the dips in alertness more if you are sleep deprived. Chronotype describes your natural tendency towards alertness or sleepiness at different times of the day – sort of like how most people probably describe themselves as either a night owl or an early riser. Timings will differ depending on your inherent chronotype. When deter-. mining your optimum sleep routine, use recommendations as a guide but also consider your chronotype. To determine yours, complete the questionnaire below.

Assessment: Morningness–Eveningness Questionnaire

- Please read each question very carefully before answering.
- Please answer each question as honestly as possible.
- Circle your answers.
- Answer ALL questions.
- Each question should be answered independently of others. Do NOT go back and check your answers.

1. What time would you get up if you were entirely free to plan your day?

5.00 – 6.29 a.m.	5
6.30 – 7.44 a.m.	4
7.45 – 9.44 a.m.	3
9.45 – 10.59 a.m.	2
11.00 – 11:59 a.m.	1
Midday – 4.59 a.m.	0

2. What time would you go to bed if you were entirely free to plan your evening?

8.00 – 8.59 p.m.	5
9.00 – 10.14 p.m.	4
10.15 p.m. – 12.29 a.m.	3
12.30 – 1.44 a.m.	2
1.45 – 2.59 a.m.	1
3.00 – 7.59 a.m.	0

3. If there is a specific time at which you have to get up in the morning, to what extent do you depend on being woken up by an alarm clock?

Not at all dependent	4
Slightly dependent	3
Fairly dependent	2
Very dependent	1

4. How easy do you find it to get up in the morning (when you are not woken up unexpectedly)?

Not at all easy	1
Not very easy	2
Fairly easy	3
Very easy	4

5. How alert do you feel during the first half-hour after you wake up in the morning?

Not at all alert	1
Slightly alert	2
Fairly alert	3
Very alert	4

6. How hungry do you feel during the first half-hour after you wake up in the morning?

Not at all hungry	1
Slightly hungry	2
Fairly hungry	3
Very hungry	4

7. During the first half-hour after you wake up in the morning, how tired do you feel?

Very tired	1
Fairly tired	2
Fairly refreshed	3
Very refreshed	4

8. If you have no commitments the next day, what time would you go to bed compared to your usual bedtime?

Seldom or never later	4
Less than one hour later	3
1–2 hours later	2
More than two hours later	1

9. You have decided to engage in some physical exercise. A friend suggests that you do this for one hour twice a week and the best time for him is between 7.00 – 8.00 a.m. Bearing in mind nothing but your own internal 'clock', how do you think you would perform?

Would be in good form	4
Would be in reasonable form	3
Would find it difficult	2
Would find it very difficult	1

10. At what time of day do you feel you become tired as a result of need for sleep?

8.00 – 8.59 p.m.	5
9.00 – 10.14 p.m.	4
10.15 p.m. – 12.44 a.m.	3
12.45 – 1.59 a.m.	2
2.00 – 3.00 a.m.	1

11. You want to be at your peak performance for a test that you know is going to be mentally exhausting and will last for two hours. You are entirely free to plan your day. Considering only your own internal 'clock', which ONE of the four testing times would you choose?

8.00 – 10.00 a.m.	4
11.00 a.m. – 1.00 p.m.	3
3.00– 5.00 p.m.	2
7.00 – 9.00 p.m.	1

12. If you got into bed at 11.00 p.m., how tired would you be?

Not at all tired	1
A little tired	2
Fairly tired	3
Very tired	4

13. For some reason, you have gone to bed several hours later than usual, but there is no need to get up at any particular time the next morning. Which ONE of the following are you most likely to do?

Will wake up at usual time, but will NOT fall back asleep	4
Will wake up at usual time and will doze thereafter	3
Will wake up at usual time but will fall asleep again	2
Will NOT wake up until later than usual	1

14. One night you have to remain awake between 4.00 – 6.00 a.m. in order to carry out a night watch. You have no commitments the next day. Which ONE of the alternatives will suite you best?

Would NOT go to bed until watch was over	1
Would take a nap before and sleep after	2
Would take a good sleep before and nap after	3
Would sleep only before watch	4

15. You have to do two hours of hard physical work. You are entirely free to plan your day and considering only your own internal 'clock' which ONE of the following times would you choose?

8.00– 10.00 a.m.	4
11.00 a.m. – 1.00 p.m.	3
3.00– 5.00 p.m.	2
7.00 – 9.00 p.m.	1

16. You have decided to engage in hard physical exercise. A friend suggests that you do this for one hour twice a week and the best time for him is 10.00 – 11.00 p.m. Bearing in mind nothing else but your own internal 'clock', how well do you think you would perform?

Would be in good form	1
Would be in reasonable form	2
Would find it difficult	3
Would find it very difficult	4

17. Suppose that you can choose your own work hours. Assume that you worked a FIVE-hour day (including breaks) and that your job was interesting and paid by results. Which FIVE CONSECUTIVE HOURS would you select?

5 hours starting between 4.00 and 7.59 a.m.	5
5 hours starting between 8.00 and 8.59 a.m.	4
5 hours starting between 9.00 a.m. and 1.59 p.m.	3
5 hours starting between 2.00 and 4.59 p.m.	2
5 hours starting between 5.00 p.m. and 3.59 a.m.	1

18. At what time of the day do you think that you reach your 'feeling best' peak?

5.00 – 7.59 a.m.	5
8.00 – 9.59 a.m.	4
10.00 a.m.– 4.59 p.m.	3
5.00 – 9.59 p.m.	2
10.00 p.m. – 4.59 a.m.	1

19. One hears about 'morning' and 'evening' types of people. Which ONE of these types do you consider yourself to be?

Definitely a 'morning' type	6
Rather more a 'morning' than an 'evening' type	4
Rather more an 'evening' than a 'morning' type	2
Definitely an 'evening' type	0

Scoring

Add up the score for all 19 questions and enter it here _____

Definite evening	16 – 30
Moderate evening	31 – 41
Intermediate	42 – 58
Moderate morning	59 – 69
Definite morning	70 – 86

Understanding your chronotype will not only help you to determine the best times for you to sleep, it will also help you to determine when you can be most productive. Schedule your most challenging mental tasks to coincide with the time of day when you feel most alert. If you are living with brain fog, there is no point making things worse by attempting difficult mental tasks when there is a natural drop in your mental alertness due to your own internal body clock.

You will fall asleep more quickly, have less disturbed and possibly even deeper sleep if you sleep when your chronotype dictates. It's hard to go against your natural tendencies, but if your job or other responsibilities and commitments make it difficult for you to align your sleep with your natural rhythm then you can try the following to minimise the impact this has:

- Never hit the snooze button, no matter what – just get up as soon as you wake up.
- Make sure that you get natural daylight as soon as possible after you wake and throughout the day.
- Start to dim artificial light from about 8 p.m.
- Exercise first thing in the morning.
- Try to keep your evenings calm and limit late nights.

Your pacemaker, the SCN, is strategically located so that it can receive signals from your optic nerve about the ambient light around you. The SCN samples the light signals that travel from your eyes along your optic nerve and uses the information about light and darkness to synchronise your internal rhythms with your external environment. It uses a circulating hormone called melatonin, which is made in and secreted from the pineal gland, to communicate its repeating signal of night and day to your brain and your body. Soon after dusk, triggered by the SCN, melatonin is rapidly released into your bloodstream. Melatonin doesn't generate sleep or have any role in the sleep process; rather it is a messenger that runs through your bloodstream like your mother's voice permeating the house when you were a kid telling you it's time for bed.

Over the course of the night, while you sleep, melatonin gradually dissipates from your system. The eventual absence of melatonin informs your brain and body that it's time to end sleep and resume wakefulness. With dawn, the release of melatonin ceases and remains shut off completely during the hours of daylight until the SCN triggers the cycle again soon after dusk. This is why managing your exposure to light – getting exposure to bright morning light each day, and dimming lights in the evening – over each twenty-four hour period is fundamental to good sleep.

The increasing pressure to sleep that you experience as the day progresses is a consequence of a build-up of a brain chemical called adenosine which requires sleep in order to be cleared from your system. Adenosine plays a critical role in the sleep–wake cycle. As it rises throughout the day you feel a building pressure to sleep.

By late evening when the circadian alerting system slackens off, your adenosine levels make you feel sleepy and the hormone melatonin is produced after dusk, calling you to sleep. While you sleep, adenosine gradually dissipates and the release of melatonin ceases in the early hours of morning.

A few hours before you wake, your circadian rhythm increases its activity, transmitting an alerting signal throughout your brain and body. The signal builds as the day progresses, reaching its peak in early afternoon. You should feel wide awake throughout the morning due to the combination of a rising circadian alerting signal and low levels of adenosine. However, if you don't get enough sleep, the adenosine won't have had time to be fully cleared from your system and you will feel groggy and tired instead of alert and refreshed. Sound familiar?

Sleep is broadly divided between two types: rapid eye movement (REM) sleep, also known as dream sleep, and non-REM sleep. If your ability to learn and remember is affected by brain fog then it could be that you are not getting sufficient of either or possibly both types of sleep. Throughout the night you will go through approximately five ninety-minute cycles. Within each of these cycles, your sleep alternates between non-REM and REM sleep, and each cycle has different proportions of each type. Earlier cycles have more non-REM sleep, but as the night progresses the proportion of REM sleep relative to non-REM sleep increases. If you sleep eight hours each night you will spend about an hour and a half in REM sleep with the highest proportion occurring in the final third of the night. You will experience your deepest sleep about three hours after you first fall asleep. If you go to bed at 11.30 p.m. and wake at 7.30 a.m., for example, you will have your longest stretch of REM sleep between about 5 and 6 a.m. If you cut your sleep short you may miss out on the benefits of REM sleep and your brain performance will suffer.

Napping

Irrespective of culture or geography, all humans experience a dip in alertness in the afternoon. Humans started to ignore this innate drive to sleep in the mid afternoon around the onset of the industrial revolution to facilitate a new, industrial style of working. Biological, neurochemical, metabolic activity plus anthropological evidence suggests that our natural propensity is for one long bout of sleep at night followed by a short bout in the afternoon. The current truth is that our sleep patterns have been contorted by industrialisation and the invention of electric light.

Is it wise to ignore this biological nudge towards a nap? Could taking a nap boost your brain performance and help to battle brain fog? Are there benefits to napping? Yes, there are and many of them directly improve domains affected in brain fog. For starters, napping recharges the brain by restoring alertness. In addition, nappers benefit from an increase in alertness in the period immediately following the nap. Furthermore, nappers benefit from extended alertness later in the day and will feel more energised and less fatigued. Napping can also improve performance, making you both faster and better. Nappers are also less likely to have accidents than their non-napping counterparts. There is evidence too that napping improves memory and learning. Power naps actually increase memory by 20 per cent for the remainder of the day and replenish your ability to learn new information. In fact, a nap can give you a 20 per cent learning advantage over someone who doesn't nap. In addition, napping or just allowing time to daydream without sleeping can increase creativity.

Whilst this evidence comes from research in the general population, not specifically people living with brain fog, given the fact that napping can reduce fatigue and boost alertness, learning, memory and processing speed it's certainly well worth giving it a try to see whether you notice any improvements. The practical tips to improve sleep later in this chapter include specific advice on napping, which is important to pay heed to as napping too late and for too long can make brain fog worse not better.

How can poor sleep contribute to brain fog?

While you are awake, your brain constantly acquires new information. This information is held temporarily in your hippocampus until the next time that you sleep. The capacity of the hippocampus is finite, which means that today's information needs to be cleared out overnight so that your hippocampus can take in new information tomorrow. As you know, your brain communicates with itself and with the rest of your body via electrical and chemical signals. *Brainwaves* are produced when masses of neurons communicate with each other by synchronised electrical pulses. Non-REM sleep is characterised by slow brainwaves interspersed with a burst of activity called spindles. During deep, non-REM sleep, slow waves and sleep spindles transfer new information from their short-term home in your hippocampus, located in your emotional brain, to a more stable permanent home in your thinking brain.

It is not possible, nor does it make sense, for you to remember and consolidate every single piece of information or experience that you encounter. Nor is it possible for you to retain every piece of information that you have ever taken in. An interesting pattern of electrical activity loops between the hippocampus and the frontal lobes ten to fifteen times during non-REM spindles. This activity most likely reflects the hippocampus checking in with the executive control unit in the frontal lobes to make information-filtering decisions about whether specific information is important or irrelevant, to be remembered or to be discarded. This means that in addition to playing a critical role in learning and memory, sleep also serves the purpose of discarding information that we don't need or information that we need to forget. Daytime napping can enhance this forgetting filtering.

Non-REM sleep allows distant regions of your brain to share the retained information with each other to strengthen new learning and consolidate new memories. Sleep in the early part of the night is better than later in the night for retaining and saving memories, so make sure you factor this into your sleep routine and get to bed before midnight.

Diane receives a lovely camellia plant as a gift. When she recalls the name of the plant shortly after learning it, she is activating her hippocampus. When she tells her husband the name of the plant the next morning – assuming she has had a good night's sleep rich in deep non-REM sleep – she is activating her neocortex. This is because the information was moved from her hippocampus to her neocortex while she slept. Sleep before learning helps you to encode or acquire new information and sleep *after* learning helps you to retain new information and consolidate memories. Sleep actually refreshes your ability to learn and make new memories.

In contrast to the slow waves and spindles of non-REM sleep, the electrical activity recorded during REM sleep is very similar to that recorded in an awake brain. During REM sleep, new information is integrated with existing information, experiences and memories. This integration updates your internal model of the world, allowing you to solve problems, gain insight and develop ideas. During the night, Diane dreams of her green-fingered mum, Helen, planting heathers. Helen is talking Diane through the process just as she did when Diane was a child. On waking, Diane realises that she will need to buy compost for acid-loving plants because camellias, like heathers, like soil with an acid pH. Her brain had presented her with a solution to a problem she hadn't even acknowledged when she was awake.

Napping that includes REM sleep can also help build connections between distantly related information. If you'd like more mornings where you wake with bright ideas and solutions, make sure you factor sufficient time for REM sleep every night.

Being deprived of just one night of sleep will impair your ability to learn and encode new information within your hippocampus. Even if you were to get a full night's sleep but were selectively deprived of non-REM sleep, the brain activity associated with learning and encoding information in the hippocampus is reduced.

To summarise, your brain needs both non-REM and REM sleep, so get your sleep at the right time, preferably beginning at some point between 8 p.m. and midnight. New information is strengthened and new memories are consolidated during non-REM sleep. New information is integrated with existing information, experiences and memories during REM sleep, allowing you to solve problems, gain insight and develop ideas.

Chronic fatigue syndrome

Antoinette: 'My life changed totally. I loved my job and going to the gym but most of all I loved being a mum. Now I spend most of my days in bed or lying on the sofa watching my little boy play. I get dizzy when I stand up and any form of activity leaves me exhausted. The gym was first to go. I thought I'd be fine at work since my job is not physical, I spend most of my days sitting at a computer doing admin and accounts. I couldn't have been more wrong; the mental exhaustion was just as bad if not worse than the physical pain and fatigue. Work stuff that I'd been doing for years on autopilot felt really challenging. It was like the wheels in my brain were trying to churn through thick mud. It was terrifying to be honest.

'At least I have a diagnosis now but back then I felt like I was caught in a nightmare I couldn't wake up from. Now my life is about choosing what activity is worth losing several days to utter exhaustion. Something simple like supermarket shopping will knock me for six. I tried online shopping but the mental challenge of that was overwhelming as well as mentally draining. It breaks my heart that I can't help my seven-year-old with his homework because my brain won't work. Now I conserve my energy for important things like going to my son's school play. It takes huge effort for me to focus and pay attention for the duration of the play to the extent that I'll need to stay in bed for a couple of days afterwards to recover.'

Antoinette has myalgic encephalomyelitis/chronic fatigue syndrome (ME/CFS), which is defined as more than six months of persistent physical and cognitive fatigue. Most patients describe their cognitive symptoms as brain fog. However, clinicians tend to refer to the slow thinking, confusion, poor concentration, difficulty focusing and cloudy thinking experienced by people with ME/CFS as mild cognitive impairment.

People with ME/CSF also experience dizziness or light-headedness on standing. The medical term for this is orthostatic intolerance. Orthostasis [from the Greek: *ortho* (upright) and *histanai* (to stand)], is a normal physiological response to counteract the fall in blood pressure that occurs when we move from lying down to standing up. Essentially, standing upright is a stressor for humans. When we stand up, gravity shifts blood volume from the upper body, including the brain, to the lower body leading to a fall in blood pressure.

In order to maintain brain blood flow, blood pressure and consciousness, your brain and your circulatory system has to compensate rapidly, so physiological compensatory mechanisms evolved as our ancestors adapted to standing and walking upright on two legs. Some people are unable to compensate for this blood volume shift. People who are chronically affected by orthostatic intolerance can feel light-headed, faint, fatigued and experience cognitive deficits on rising from lying down to standing or when standing for long periods such as waiting in line or taking a shower. The only way for them to alleviate their symptoms is to sit or lie down.

Brain scans of people with ME/CFS indicate that their brains need greater activation to complete difficult mental tasks than their healthy counterparts. People with ME/CFS have deficits in attention, concentration, working memory and the speed and efficiency with which they can process information. They then perceive these issues as an exaggerated mental fatigue. Stress, including physical exercise, mental challenges and orthostatic stress make their brain fog worse. Most treatments for ME/CFS have focused on the physical fatigue rather the brain fog symptoms. Cognitive behavioural therapy (CBT) and graded exercise therapy have been used effectively to treat people with ME/CFS, which is a good indication that it may also help with the experience of brain fog, although more research is needed to confirm this.

Practical tips to improve sleep

Any plan to improve your sleep needs to take account of the wider context of your life and habits as well as the environment in which you sleep.

Julie has been experiencing brain fog symptoms for several years. Together with her GP, she has ruled out any underlying medical conditions and hormonal issues. She has a demanding job. In order to keep her head above water she leads a healthy lifestyle, eats a balanced diet and exercises regularly. Despite this, she says she never wakes up feeling refreshed. In fact, she says that her brain feels decidedly muggy in the morning. She has to drag herself out of the bed every morning and feels sleepy throughout the day. She loves to exercise because it gives her energy but then, rather maddeningly, when it comes time to go to bed she is totally hyped and simply can't relax. It's like her alertness is topsy-turvy – she is alert when she needs to sleep and sleepy when she needs to be alert.

Julie kept a sleep diary and, over time, established that she functions best on eight hours sleep. Monday to Friday she needs to get up at 7 a.m. so she now regularly goes to bed at 11 p.m. Of course she has the occasional late night when out with friends but she tries to limit them to once every couple of weeks. She still sees her friends as much as she did before; they just meet earlier in the evening, often straight after work. Julie makes a conscious effort not to schedule a late night with her girlfriends ahead of a day where she needs her brain to be sharp. In addition, she incorporates a nap before or after a girl's night to pre-empt or repay the inevitable sleep debt she will accrue from staying out late.

Julie has cut back on alcohol because she noticed that she doesn't sleep as soundly when she has had a few drinks. She still drinks at social occasions but she no longer drinks at home. She never goes to the gym in the late evening anymore because she realised she felt far too hyped up afterwards to be able to sleep. Now she gets up at the same time every day and goes to the gym first thing in the morning on Saturdays and Sundays. She also incorporates aerobic exercise into her routine by cycling rather than driving to work, giving her the added bonus of more exposure to natural daylight.

Julie has also started to dim the lights in her living room from about 8 p.m. onwards. She turns off overhead and other bright lighting. At 10 p.m. Julie switches off the heating, the TV and other devices and has a hot bath or listens to music, an audio book or relaxing podcasts instead. Julie admits she found this to be the toughest change to make but is glad she has persevered because she has noticed a huge reduction in her brain fog symptoms.

1. Quantity, quality and regularity

The best time to go to bed is very individual and depends on your chronotype, when you need to wake and how much sleep you need.

The best way to determine your optimum bedtime and sleep duration is to keep a sleep log. Over time you may notice that you feel more refreshed on waking on certain days. How much sleep did you have that night and what time did you go to bed? Is there a pattern emerging that might help you to determine what works for you? Even the smallest of improvements or dis-improvements in how you feel on waking can help to point you in the right directions. You may also need to look more closely at whether your daily schedule, including your working hours, are running counter to your natural rhythms.

To determine your bedtime, work back from the time that you have to get up each morning. Initially aim to spend approximately eight hours in bed and adjust this accordingly based on how you feel in the morning. You may feel better on more or less hours spent in bed. Try to avoid alarm clocks. If you calculate your best bed time by working backwards from the time that you need to wake, you should wake naturally for work instead of being rudely awakened by an alarm.

If you are getting fewer than the recommended hours of sleep because you regularly go to bed after midnight, you may be depriving your brain of the time to carry out the important activities of non-REM sleep. Conversely, if you regularly cut short your sleep by getting up ultra-early you may be depriving your brain of a large proportion of the time needed to carry out the activities of REM sleep.

Stick to a schedule. That means going to bed and getting up at the same time every day regardless of whether it is the weekend or your day off. Your circadian rhythm works best with regular sleep habits. Also bear in mind that your circadian rhythms can change across your lifespan so you may need to adjust your sleep schedule accordingly. What worked for you in your twenties and thirties may no longer work in your fifties or sixties. Rather than aligning your sleep time with that of your partner or 'on average' guidelines, it's far better to pay attention to your body and work with your own personal feelings of alertness and drowsiness. It is well worth developing a wind-down routine for the evenings, as Julie did.

2. Manage exposure to light

For billions of years the sun has provided light during the day and virtually no light at night. Almost all life forms have developed a circadian rhythm which is kept at twenty-hours by the daily cycle of light and dark. Electric light, which has only been widely available for about one hundred years disrupts the circadian rhythm, the sleep–wake cycle, hormone regulation and core body temperature. Our use of electric light means that we have too much light at night which makes it difficult for the brain to detect true dark. In addition, we often spend huge portions of our days indoors with inadequate exposure to natural daylight. Making a conscious effort to manage your exposure to light can help to reset your natural rhythms, improve sleep and also restore hormonal balance all of which will help to combat brain fog.

Electric light

You need to carefully manage your light exposure to optimise your sleep. If 11 p.m. is your ideal bed time, from about 8 p.m. lower or dim the lighting in the room where you spend your evenings. After dinner, get in the habit of turning off or dimming overhead lights completely and use low lighting such as side lamps.

Avoid turning on bright light in the bathroom last thing at night to avoid waking up your brain with bright light that mimics daylight. Invest in a dimmer switch. Alternatively, consider altering your bedroom routine so that brushing your teeth under bright lights in the bathroom is not the very last thing that you do before you go to bed.

Make sure your bedroom is as dark as possible at night, as this will help you to sleep. Avoid switching on ultra-bright lights should you wake during the night, but make sure you have a safe route to the bathroom. Low-level night-lights can guide the way; you can get battery operated adhesive ones, or a bedside torch would work too.

Natural light

Make sure that you get exposure to natural light for at least thirty minutes every day. If you can, try to get exposure to morning sunlight; open the shutters or curtains as soon as possible after waking. If you live in a part of the world where winter mornings are dark, turn on the lights in your bedroom when you wake. The white light will help to mimic day light.

Blue light

Artificial blue light is emitted from digital devices and from LED lighting. This blue light wavelength is beneficial during the day because it boosts attention, reaction time and mood. However, blue light is disruptive at night-time because it keeps you awake. Avoid blue-light exposure for an hour before sleep and altogether in the bedroom. If you wake in the night, don't be tempted to reach for your phone or laptop because the device's blue light will wake your brain and make it difficult to get back to sleep. If at all possible, leave your devices charging anywhere in the house other than in your bedroom. Aim to make your bedroom a technology-free zone. Get yourself a traditional alarm clock to check the time and wake you up. This will prevent you falling down the rabbit hole of checking the time on your phone, which not only exposes you to blue light but also increases the risk of clicking on email or social media notifications.

Use software/apps on your devices that gradually desaturate the harmful blue LED light as the evening progresses. If you plan to go to bed at 11 p.m. then turn off the TV and other devices at 10 p.m. and switch to a more relaxing activity such as listening to music or reading a print book beside a side lamp. Consider using aromas such as natural aromatherapy candles or diffusers if these help you to relax. Given that most of us now have access to TV shows on demand there is no need to stay up late watching something that you can just as easily watch early the next evening without interrupting your sleep schedule.

3. Find the right temperature

Controlling the temperature in your environment is as important as controlling the light. Your core body temperature rises and falls by a small amount over each twenty-four-hour period in a pattern that is related to your sleep cycle. As a cue to sleep, your core temperature drops with drowsiness as you come towards the sleep phase of your sleep–wake cycle. In order to initiate sleep your core body temperature actually needs to drop by 1 degree Celsius. Once your core temperature dips below a threshold, heat-sensitive cells send a message to the

SCN spurring it on to release melatonin. So both light and temperature independently but in synchrony dictate your night-time melatonin levels shaping your ideal bed time. As you come close to waking, your core temperature warms up again.

Your hypothalamus is responsible for maintaining your core temperature and returning it to homeostasis should it deviate from the healthy window. This is a critical function since both high (e.g. 42°C) and low temperatures (e.g. 35°C) can lead to brain damage and death. Fever, exercise, digestion, alcohol, drugs or an underactive thyroid can alter your core temperature. When your central nervous system senses a change in your internal temperature, it sends messages to your hypothalamus. Informed that your internal temperature is becoming too high or too low, your hypothalamus sends messages to your nervous system, glands, muscles and organs to take action to get your temperature back within its optimum range. For example, if you become too hot or too cold during the night your sleep may be disrupted by sweating or shivering. Managing external factors that influence your temperature before and while you sleep will help you to fall asleep and stay asleep throughout the night.

It's easier to fall asleep in a cool room rather than a hot room. Turn the heat off or down in your home an hour before bedtime. Aim for a sleep-inducing bedroom temperature of about 16–18°C, assuming you will be using a duvet and wearing pyjamas.

To help cool your core body temperature, consider taking a hot bath thirty minutes before bedtime. I know this sounds counterintuitive, but when you get out of the bath your dilated blood vessels help radiate heat out to the surface of your skin and away from the core, lowering your core body temperature. If you don't have a bath in your home or don't fancy a hot bath, selectively warming your hands or feet by about 0.5°C will encourage blood away from your core to your extremities, thereby reducing your core temperature.

If you find yourself overheating due to menopause or pregnancy, consider wearing pyjamas that wick away moisture. Keep a spare pair of pyjamas, towels, pillowcases and sheets close to your bed so that you can dry off and change without having to hunt them down in the middle of the night.

4. Improve your sleep environment

Your bedroom should be a haven for sleep. Ideally, sex is the only other activity that should take place there. If your living arrangements permit, try to make your bedroom a haven for sleep, avoiding dual-purpose use such as home office or watching TV. Many teen and kids' bedrooms are dual purpose, filled with toys and consoles and often desks for study. With more and more people working from home, many adults have had to create a work space in their bedroom. If space limitations make this unavoidable, find ways to transform the room from day use to sleep haven by shutting down and removing devices and tidying toys and study or work materials away. There are lots of ingenious storage solutions that will allow you to do this.

Remember, sleep is not a luxury. Sleep is essential if you want your brain and body to work properly. If your sleeping environment is less than ideal, weigh up the financial cost of revamping your bedroom against the personal cost of brain fog. Whatever the current trend in bedroom decor, calming colours without patterns are the most conducive to sleep. Invest in curtains or shutters that completely block out light.

Remove clutter from your sleeping space. Clutter triggers the release of the stress hormone cortisol which will interfere with your ability to sleep. Keep your room tidy and remove anything that doesn't need to be there, particularly items that make you feel stressed or anxious. Find somewhere else to store them or dump them completely. Keep dust in your bedroom under control and change your bedclothes regularly. Invest in good quality bed clothes. Good-quality cotton sheets help me to stay cool if my body overheats at night. Don't forget that pillows and mattresses need to be changed too. Do what you can to eliminate noises or smells that prevent you from sleeping.

5. Nap

Consider responding to your biological rhythm by taking a nap at a regular time each day to see whether this reduces any of your brain fog symptoms. Timing and duration of naps are critical. Naps are best taken about six to eight hours after waking and, as a general rule, no later than 3 p.m. Everyone is different but it is important to time it so that it doesn't interfere with your night-time sleep.

Light sleepers or people with insomnia should leave seven to eight hours between their nap and normal bed time, while others can leave three to four hours. Ideally naps should be for less than twenty minutes or for a full sleep cycle (i.e. ninety minutes). Ten-minute naps are most beneficial in terms of reducing sleepiness and improving cognitive performance. I've been known to take the occasional ten-minute nap around 2 p.m. while writing this book if I've felt my eyelids drooping. Napping for forty to sixty minutes will mean you wake up in the middle of slow-wave sleep leading to sleep inertia, which means you will wake feeling tired, disoriented and sluggish.

In later life, melatonin release reaches its peak earlier in the evening, nudging us towards an earlier bedtime. You may struggle to stay awake in the evening but if you inadvertently nod off mid-evening it counts as a nap, which unfortunately dilutes sleep pressure to the extent that you may struggle to get to sleep when you eventually go to bed.

As you get older, your circadian clock also tends to wake you up earlier in the morning. If you continually refuse to take account of the changing rhythms and pressures of your body, you will push yourself further and further into sleep debt. You can respond to the pressure to sleep earlier. Alternatively, sleep researcher Matthew Walker suggests tailoring your light exposure to gain greater control over age-related changes in your circadian rhythm by getting more exposure to natural light in the afternoons, which will push out the time at which melatonin is released.

Another option is to consider napping strategically to minimise your brain fog. For example, you could use napping prophylactically by taking a nap in the early afternoon to ward off unintentional napping too close to bedtime or, like Julie, in advance when you know you have a late night ahead. You may also find an emergency nap beneficial in response to overwhelming tiredness or fatigue, to prevent accidents (you are seven times more likely to make an error when you are sleepy), or to combat drowsy driving.

Drowsy driving accidents occur most frequently during the afternoon dip in your circadian rhythm and between the hours of midnight and 6 a.m. when your brain expects to be asleep. It is not possible to drive safely on insufficient sleep because your attention is impaired, your reaction time slows, you are more likely to take risks and your ability to make decisions is disrupted. Drowsy driving claims almost as many lives as drunk driving. Driving is a cognitively demanding task. Cognitive resources become depleted when you do the same task for extended periods, so your performance decreases the longer you spend driving, with the number of errors you make increasing progressively.

The best advice for maintaining good sleep hygiene is to avoid caffeine. However, when it comes to combatting drowsy driving caffeine can come in useful. If you find yourself becoming drowsy while driving, pull into a rest area as soon as possible, drink a cup of coffee and take a short nap, no more than twenty minutes. Any longer than that and you risk going into a deep sleep which can be very difficult to wake from and can leave you 'sleep drunk' and more tired than before you napped. A fifteen-minute nap reduces the levels of the sleep pressure chemical adenosine. It takes about twenty minutes for the caffeine to go through your system so you wake just as the caffeine, which will have less adenosine to deal with, kicks in. The caffeine nap is a useful quick fix to restore alertness and avoid accidents.

6. Things to avoid before bedtime

It is important to plan your evening so that it is not overly stimulating close to bedtime, as this may make it difficult to fall and stay asleep. Eliminate stimulants such as alcohol, caffeine and cigarettes completely if possible and avoid exercise and any stressful or anxiety-inducing activities in the evening time.

Alcohol

Avoid alcohol close to bedtime. Alcohol is a sedative but don't be fooled by the fact it makes you feel sleepy – it does not induce natural sleep. Alcohol disrupts sleep with mini awakenings, meaning sleep is not continuous and therefore not restorative. After a few hours, alcohol acts as a stimulant that interferes with the quality of your sleep. In fact, it supresses REM sleep, depriving you of dream sleep and its associated benefits. Ditch the nightcap altogether and, if you do drink, try to keep it to early evening (e.g. with dinner). Limit consumption to two units or fewer and avoid binge-drinking large quantities of alcohol.

Caffeine

Caffeine is a psychoactive stimulant. You feel stimulated and alert because caffeine dampens the effect of the sleep-pressure chemical adenosine. Caffeine doesn't get rid of adenosine from your system, though, nor does it magically pay off your sleep debt. Caffeine just blocks the 'I'm sleepy' signal, tricking you into feeling alert. You still need to sleep. The sleep debt continues to build. Caffeine persists in your system for quite some time after consumption. It can take five to seven hours to clear just half of it. As you get older, the time it takes your brain and body to process and remove caffeine from your system increases. Try not to consume caffeine within five hours of bedtime and remember that even decaffeinated coffee may contain up to 3 per cent caffeine.

Smoking

Nicotine is a stimulant. If your plan is to cut down on the number of cigarettes that you smoke gradually rather than go cold turkey, avoid nicotine, including patches and gum, for at least an hour before bedtime.

Eating and drinking

Don't eat late at night and avoid foods (e.g. high-fat foods, spicy foods, foods high in salt, alcohol, carbonated drinks) that promote heartburn, which is more likely to occur if you lie down soon after eating. Avoid foods and drinks that contain caffeine (e.g. chocolate, tea, coffee, soft drinks) for five to six hours before bed. Avoid drinking too much water before bedtime; spreading your water consumption throughout the day instead will keep you hydrated and will help to cut down night-time trips to the bathroom.

Exercise

Exercise is brilliant for promoting sleep so make sure that you get exercise every day, preferably in the morning, afternoon or early evening. Avoid exercise altogether within three hours of your optimum bedtime because it stimulates your brain and elevates your core temperature, both of which make it difficult to sleep.

Stress

Dealing with stressful issues, worries or anxiety-inducing thoughts in the evening time, particularly close to your bedtime, is a recipe for wakefulness. Set aside time in the morning or during the day to deal with these issues to avoid them keeping you awake at night. Chapter 6 is packed with tips for managing stress.

7. Minimise the impact of shift work and jet lag

Shift work and jet lag disrupt normal circadian rhythms and are associated with brain fog. One study suggests that 10 years of shift work resulted in a loss equivalent to 6.5 years of age-related decline in cognitive function. Recovery of cognitive function after giving up shift work took at least five years. The National Sleep Foundation recommends the following to minimise sleep disruption and improve sleep quality for night-shift workers:

- Keep the same sleep and wake times every day to regulate your circadian rhythm.
- If you must rotate your shifts, try to rotate clockwise, going from day shift to evening shift to night shift. Avoid the reverse or rotating without a pattern.
- To prepare for a new shift, gradually adjust sleep and wake times over the three days prior to your shift. For example, if rotating clockwise this means delaying your bedtime and wake time by two hours each night.

If you are flying long haul, to minimise jet lag:

- Where possible, choose a flight that allows early evening arrival and stay up until 10 p.m. local time.
- If you must take a nap during the day, limit it to early afternoon.
- Avoid alcohol and caffeine.
- Get out in the daylight as it will help to regulate your biological clock. Staying indoors worsens jet lag.

8. Managing medical conditions and medications

If you are kept awake by the symptoms of a chronic condition, it is worth speaking to a member of your medical team to learn about ways to minimise symptoms and improve your sleep quality. Sleep loss and sleep disturbances also increase your sensitivity to pain which, in its own right, can lead to brain fog.

Medication

If you take medications and experience difficulty falling asleep, staying asleep, daytime drowsiness or other disruptions in your sleep patterns, it might be worth a visit to your doctor to see whether the medication is the culprit. Some heart, blood pressure and asthma medications can interfere with sleep, as can over-the-counter cold, flu and headache tablets. The chemicals in these medications don't always affect everyone in the same way.

When I started taking a new migraine medication I experienced terrible trouble getting to sleep and developed very vivid dreams. I really didn't want to stop taking the medication as it had significantly reduced the number and severity of my migraines. When my neurologist asked me how I was getting on with the new medication, I mentioned my sleep issues. He suggested taking the meds first thing in the morning instead of last thing at night. I did this and, while I continued to have vivid dreams, I no longer had difficulty getting to sleep at night.

Don't stop prescribed medications or change the times that you take them of your own accord; always consult with your doctor to find alternatives that don't impact on your sleep.

If you have been prescribed sleeping pills it is possible that they are at the root of your brain fog. Sleeping pills do not induce natural restorative sleep. In fact, next day you will feel groggy, forgetful and your reaction times will be impaired. The electrical activity of sleeping-pill-induced 'sleep' is missing the largest, deepest brain waves that are qualitatively different to the brain waves observed during natural sleep. While natural deep sleep helps to embed memory traces in the brain, some sleeping pills actually weaken connections already formed during learning, connections that should be strengthened during sleep. Memories are therefore lost rather than saved.

Sleeping pills target the same systems in the brain as alcohol. They are sedatives that stop the brain cells in the higher regions of your brain from firing. Sadly 'rebound insomnia' means that when you stop taking sleeping pills you may be left with worse sleeping problems than you had in the first instance. I will reiterate here, though, that you should never stop taking prescription medication of your own accord. Speak to your prescribing doctor about your medication and discuss alternative behavioural methods to improve your natural sleep.

Insomnia

Symptoms of insomnia include brain fog, fatigue, low energy and irritability. If you experience difficulty sleeping three times a week for at least three months you meet the criteria for a diagnosis of insomnia. While insomnia is a recognised sleep disorder, it is important to note that if you do get a diagnosis it doesn't mean that your insomnia will be persistent because insomnia can be transient or episodic.

Insomnia affects more women than men and more older people than younger people. Difficulty getting to sleep is called sleep onset insomnia. Falling asleep but waking frequently during sleep is called short sleep insomnia. For sleep to be restorative both quantity and quality matter. An individual with short sleep insomnia could sleep for ten hours but not cycle through five stages of sleep due to frequent waking.

Insomnia is strongly linked to stress, anxiety and depression. People with anxiety are at increased risk for developing insomnia. The anxiety doesn't cause the insomnia; it just increases the likelihood that it will occur. Insomnia is often precipitated by life's stressors – grief, money worries, relationship problems, work challenges. It can also be perpetuated by certain behaviours including irregular sleep habits, technology use and low levels of physical activity. One of the first lines of treatment is to develop good sleep habits also referred to as sleep hygiene, as outlined above.

Cognitive behavioural therapy for insomnia (CBT-I) also works well as does treating any underlying conditions such as depression and anxiety. Building on good sleep hygiene, a CBT-I therapist works with the patient over several weeks to eradicate bad sleep habits and address anxieties associated with sleeping. One form of CBT-I actually involves restricting the amount of time spent in bed to as little as six hours, thereby allowing adenosine and stronger sleep pressure to build. Under this heavy pressure to sleep, the individual may fall asleep easier and regain psychological confidence in their ability to get to sleep. Once the patient has developed a regular habit of self-generating sleep under this strong sleep pressure, the amount of time they spend in bed is gradually increased to recommended levels.

If your insomnia persists despite improving your sleep habits, then speak to your doctor about other behavioural treatments or request a referral to a sleep specialist.

Key chapter takeaways

- Work with, not against, your natural rhythm.
- Napping boosts brain function.
- Quantity and quality matter when it comes to sleep.
- Stick to a sleep schedule.
- Soak up natural daylight, sleep in the dark and beware of blue light.
- Cool your core.
- Shape a sleep haven.
- Nap early for ninety minutes or less than twenty.
- Avoid stimulants.
- Chat to your doctor about medical conditions and medications.
- Sleeping tablets do not induce natural sleep.
- Try behavioural methods to tackle insomnia.
- If all else fails, seek a sleep specialist.

Get ready for the 30-day plan

I've compiled a list of practical things that you can do in advance of starting the 30-day plan. Think of these activities as you would the things you do in advance of the first day back at school.

1. Sleeping quarters upgrade

a. Put fresh bedclothes on your bed.

b. Pick up any clothes off the floor, put soiled clothes in the laundry basket and fold clean clothes into drawers or the wardrobe.

c. Remove jewellery, creams or other bits and bobs from your nightstand.

d. Vacuum the floor and dust the surfaces.

e. Remove technology other than lights from your bedroom. If anything can't be removed then unplug it.

If you live with fatigue, chronic pain or any other issue that makes any of the above tasks particularly arduous, call in the troops (family or friends) to give you a hand or do it for you.

2. Dispatch devices

a. Identify a place other than your bedroom to charge your devices. Move all your charges there now.

b. Install software/apps on your devices (phones, tablets, laptop) that gradually desaturate the harmful blue LED light as the evening progresses.

3. Deal with disruptions

a. Revisit the sleep disruption assessment that you completed earlier in this chapter. Are there any barriers to sleep that you could take action on now?

b. If a streetlamp outside your bedroom window makes it tough to sleep, consider buying blackout curtains or blinds. They are relatively inexpensive and widely available online and in stores like IKEA, and some of them double as sound absorbers too.

c. If noise is the issue take some time to consider if there is anything you can do about the noise itself. It could be something simple like putting your dishwasher on an hour earlier in the evening so that noise won't prevent you from sleeping. If noise from neighbours is the issue speak to them nicely, appealing to their better nature, and explain as calmly as you can what you need. Would placing your bed in another part of the room help? Would swapping rooms help if your living room is in a quieter location than your bedroom? If all else fails, get some ear plugs.

4. Wake-up call

If you need an alarm to wake up and have a traditional alarm clock then move it into your bedroom and set the alarm for your optimal wake time. If you don't have an old-school alarm clock, consider investing in one. Though this is not essential since over the course of the 30-day plan, if you stick to a regular bedtime, you will start to wake naturally at your scheduled time. You can, of course, continue to set an alarm if it helps you feel less stressed or less anxious.

Change: Stress

What is stress?

Experiencing severe or prolonged stress can negatively impact on your overall health and can be particularly harmful to your central nervous system, affecting not just how your brain works but also how you behave. Chronic stress doesn't just cause brain fog, it can also lead to or increase your risk of mental ill-health and physical illness and disease.

You will probably be aware that the stress response evolved to allow us humans to fight or flee when faced with a threat. It is a product of natural selection that ensures you have the best chance of survival in that instant while also making sure that your body returns to optimum conditions for health after the threat has passed.

Stress in the short term can actually enhance your memory function but poorly managed chronic stress and persistently high levels of stress hormones can contribute to brain fog by interfering with your ability to think clearly and impairing your ability to learn and to remember.

The word 'stress' tends to be used in everyday conversation to mean the thing that makes you feel uptight or tense, the physiological changes that occur in your body, as well as the psychological and neurobiological aspects of the phenomenon. In a sense, stress is all of these things. In order to understand and manage stress it is helpful to distinguish each aspect.

Let's call the thing that stresses you the stressor. We perceive a stressor as dangerous or threatening. A stressor can also be a barrier preventing us reaching a goal or stopping us from doing what we need, want or had planned to do. Stressors can be something mundane like being stuck in a traffic jam, life-changing like losing your job or catastrophic like rape or a tsunami. Not all stressors are bad. Some stressors, like competition in sport or taking exams, can have a positive impact. We tend to think of the threat that activates the stress response as something external to ourselves, the proverbial tiger or assailant in a dark alley, but illness, injury, pain, prolonged exertion and extremes of temperature can also lead to the release of stress hormones. You can also experience psychological stress when you perceive that the demands placed on you exceed your ability to cope. For example, during the global COVID-19 pandemic, many parents were continually stressed because they felt unequipped to work from home and also home-school their kids.

A stressor kicks off a sequence of coordinated neurophysiological events in your brain and your body. These events allow you to respond to the stressor (fight or flee) and then return your body to homeostasis, which is the optimum condition that has been disturbed by the stressor. Let's call this neurophysiological response the stress response.

The stress response was originally researched in the context of acute illness and injury. With time, scientists came to understand that the neurophysiological stress response could also be activated by psychological states, such as perceived loss of control, the absence of predictability and the loss of social support. Something that became very evident to all of us during the pandemic, when so much was beyond our control and many didn't have access to their usual social support network.

With psychological stress, it doesn't even matter whether the stressor is real or imagined, as once the individual believes that a stressor or potential stressor is something that they feel unequipped to cope with, the neurophysiological stress response will be activated. Psychological stress can also be activated when you think in a negative or exaggerated way about something from your past, something going on in your life now or some scenario from an imagined future.

Different stressors activate the stress response for different people. It really is very individual and related to how a person appraises or perceives the stressful situation. First, we evaluate the threat to determine whether it is real and assess its seriousness. Then we look to our own resources and assess whether we have what it takes to meet the challenge posed by the stressor. The highest level of stress will be experienced if we decide that we cannot deal effectively with a stressor that we perceive as dangerous. Different people will make different determinations in the same set of circumstances, whereby one individual might be highly stressed and another not at all stressed or may even feel excitement. Some people jump out of aeroplanes for fun and others are terrified of flying.

A study that looked at coping with long-term stress in business executives found that some of the executives became ill and others did not. The executives who remained healthy felt in control and viewed their stressors as challenges that they met head on. The executives who became ill tended to avoid the stressors or become anxious about them. While one individual may perceive a potentially stressful situation drastically differently to the next, some things, such as a life-threatening injury or a violent encounter, will reliably activate the stress response.

Stressors can take many forms, not all of which have negative outcomes. Common stressors include: getting divorced, getting married, having a baby, losing a loved one, starting a new job, becoming unemployed, going on holiday, working long hours, learning a new hobby, giving a talk, commuting, fears, perfectionism and worrying about future events. What one person interprets as a stressor another can interpret as exciting or something to look forward to. Either way the physiological stress response is activated. If this response fails to shut down and becomes chronic your cognitive function is likely to suffer.

Are you stressed?

Learning to recognise the signs and symptoms of stress will help you to take action to reduce its harmful effects and minimise the likelihood that stress will become chronic.

Assessment: Signs of Stress

Tick any that apply to you.

Lost your sense of humour? ☐
Stress can steal your sense of humour, robbing you of your ability to see the funny side of life. Laughter is the ultimate stress buster and humour helps you to cope with the unthinkable. Laughter actually reduces levels of the stress hormone cortisol.

Is forgetfulness one of your brain fog symptoms? ☐
Absentmindedness is a common sign of stress. Stress interferes with the ability to learn and remember and can make you forget to do things in the future, like taking regular medication or meeting a friend for lunch. Concentration and sleep can also be impacted by stress. Sleep disturbance and impaired concentration can then, in turn, impact negatively on memory function.

All work and no play? ☐
If stress is prolonged or chronic it can trick you into narrowing focus to the extent that you fail to set aside time for physical exercise or other leisure activities such as hobbies, music, art or reading, or even just socialising with family and friends.

Unhealthy eating habits? ☐
Stress can lead to overeating and unhealthy food choices. In the short term, it can suppress appetite but in the longer term if stress becomes chronic and is left unmanaged, cortisol can increase your appetite and your motivation to eat. Caffeinated drinks and foods high in sugar can contribute to stress by ramping up your amygdala.

Not sleeping or sleeping fitfully? ☐
Stress can make it difficult to fall asleep and stay asleep. When your body is in balance, cortisol is secreted into your blood in a predictable twenty-four-hour rhythm. Chronic stress can interfere with this natural rhythm. Anyone who has experienced disturbed sleep due to stress

knows what it's like to be woken in the middle of the night with too much cortisol sloshing around, feeling anxious and wired, only to fall asleep in the early morning unable to rouse yourself when your alarm goes off because your cortisol levels are depleted.

Feeling lonely? ☐

When stress is overwhelming it is very tempting to shut others out of our lives, perhaps because we feel we need time alone to think or even because we feel hostile to others. We might also avoid friends and family in order not to inflict our stress-induced crankiness or irritability on them. The effort required to be with other people can feel like added

	Never	Once a month	Once a week
No sense of humour			
Forgetful or absentminded			
All work and no play			
Unhealthy eating habits			
Not sleeping or sleeping fitfully			
Feeling lonely or isolated			
Headaches			
Feeling irritable			
Tense muscles			
Feeling tired or fatigued			
Bored			
Depressed			
Short-tempered, angry or hostile			
Worried			
Anxious			
Feelings of panic			
Upset stomach			
Restless, itchy, uncomfortable in your own skin			

stress, so we end up isolating ourselves at the very time that we should be seeking social support. But this can actually make things worse and have profound effects on our physical, mental and brain health. Staying socially engaged is critical for healthy brain function.

Assessment: Stress Frequency

Indicate the frequency at which you experience the signs/symptoms of stress in the table to get a sense of the impact of stress on your life and behaviour.

	2–3 times a week	Every day	1–2 times a day	All the time

Assessment: Stress Log

If you suspect that poorly managed, chronic stress is contributing to your brain fog, keep a log of any stress that you experience. This will help you to understand your enemy so that you can better control it.

If you don't experience any stress, leave the log blank. If you have more than one stressful experience in any day, note down each one. This will help you to identify patterns.

Duration: The total time from when you began feeling stressed to when you returned to feeling calm.

Stressor: The thing, thought, person, situation, event, etc., that led to your feelings of stress.

Location: Where you were, e.g. at work, home, supermarket, motorway.

Activity: What you were doing at the time, e.g. dealing with a customer, solving a problem, arguing, parenting, thinking, trying to sleep.

Level: The level your stress reached at its peak: 1 = mild, 2 = moderate, 3 = strong, 4 = severe.

Regularity: Indicate the number of times you have felt stressed by this particular stressor in the past month.

Coping strategy: Indicate any strategy you used to cope with the experience.

Day	Time	Duration	Stressor	Location	Activity	Level	Regularity	Strategy

Your stress sweet spot

Encountering stressors that elicit the stress response can help you to learn from experience and progress through life; stressful experiences can even motivate you to attain your goals and meet daily challenges. Well-managed stress will support you through challenge and change, helping you to adapt to your environment, making you more resilient and better equipped for whatever life throws at you.

Stress is not inherently bad; in fact, the total absence of stress is not something to strive for. Too little stress is associated with boredom, disengagement and can ultimately lead to depression. Furthermore, an under-stimulated brain will lose brain volume and brain function. The key lies in finding your stress sweet spot where your brain can grow and benefit from challenge that pushes you beyond your comfort zone while maintaining homeostasis. This means embracing challenge but managing the associated stress response so that it is proportionate to the stressor and doesn't become prolonged and interfere with your overall health, wellbeing and brain function.

Anxiety

Anxiety is a normal response to stressors. It's important to distinguish between anxiety that serves a purpose, such as when it alerts you to danger and helps you prepare and pay attention, and anxiety that interferes with your ability to function.

The amygdala is a tiny structure located in the emotional brain. It plays a key role in fear and the fight or flight response. When stress becomes chronic, the growth of new brain connections in the amygdala is increased which can give rise to stronger fear memories and heightened fear responses. In parallel, the growth of new brain connections is suppressed in the frontal lobes which are responsible for overriding an irrational or overexuberant amygdala. Taken together, this means that when we are stressed we learn to be more afraid when there is no need to be. It also means that we can become less rational and less able to detect when we are safe. This could, over time, lead to an anxiety disorder. Brain fog is often a symptom of an anxiety disorder. Because symptoms of chronic stress can develop slowly over time it can be difficult to determine when things have gone too far. If your stress has been prolonged and is interfering with your ability to carry out everyday activities it may be worth speaking to a health professional to rule out an anxiety disorder or to receive appropriate treatment and support should one be identified.

Anxiety disorders differ from normal or proportionate feelings. They involve excessive fear or anxiety and can cause people to avoid situations in ways that affect their jobs, schoolwork, exam grades, performance and relationships. Generally speaking, for a person to be diagnosed with an anxiety disorder, their fear or anxiety must interfere with their ability to function normally and be disproportionate to the situation. This is very different to anxious feelings that are proportionate to a worrying event or situation.

Anxiety is the most common mental health condition in the world with one in three women and one in five men experiencing it at some point in their lives. Fear is associated with the fight or flight response to an immediate and present threat (stressor). In contrast, anxiety is the anticipation of a future concern, thinking about something that might happen. It's often associated with muscle tension and avoidance behaviour – for example, not going on holiday to avoid the anxiety of flying. There are several types of anxiety disorders. For a diagnosis, most have to have been present for at least six months and interfere with your ability to carry out daily activities.

Generalised anxiety disorder is characterised by persistent and excessive worry, often about everyday things. It can be accompanied by symptoms such as muscle tension, feeling restless and/or on edge and having trouble concentrating. Other anxiety related disorders include panic disorder, various phobias, social anxiety disorder and separation anxiety disorder. Anxiety is also prominent in obsessive compulsive disorder (OCD) and post-traumatic stress disorder (PTSD).

Depression

Anxiety and depression are closely linked. One can lead to the other or they can occur at the same time with each reinforcing the other. Just as feeling nervous or anxious sometimes is normal, so too is feeling sad and apathetic. However, these feelings are often a consequence of unhealthy life choices such as poor diet, lack of exercise and poor sleep. At other times, there is no apparent cause and the symptoms are deep, debilitating, distressing and need professional intervention.

When you are healthy, your rational prefrontal cortex keeps your emotional amygdala in check. In people with depression, the electrical activity is less active in the thinking prefrontal cortex and more active in the amygdala than in people without depression. The ENIGMA (Enhancing NeuroImaging Genetics through Meta-Analysis) study – a global alliance of over 1,400 scientists across 43 countries studying the human brain in health and disease – compared the brains of people with and without depression. In those with long-lasting or severe depression, the study found that the hippocampus, the amygdala and other related structures were slightly smaller than the same structures in people without depression. Given that the same structures in people with milder depression or one-off cases of depression were not smaller, the ENIGMA researchers propose that severe or long-lasting depression is the cause of the damage rather than the alternative possibility that people with depression have smaller structures to begin with.

Patricia has lived with severe depression most of her adult life. Thankfully, she has a loving and supportive family who help her out, especially when she struggles with making decisions or when she experiences other issues with her executive functioning. Her memory is affected too. It pains her greatly when her husband and kids talk about family memories that she simply has no recollection of. She finds it hard to understand how she can't recall these memories from her own life.

Given the findings of the ENIGMA study, it's possible that the autobiographical memory deficits that she experiences are a consequence of a reduction in the size of the hippocampus. Patricia also finds it difficult to learn new things and this too could be a consequence of a smaller hippocampus, as it is critical to both learning and memory. Unfortunately, this difficulty in learning new things has also impaired Patricia's treatment as she has struggled to learn new ways of thinking that would aid her recovery.

The type of impairments that Patricia and others with depression experience can often persist after a depressive episode has resolved.

In major depressive disorder, brain fog symptoms can include problems with attention, processing speed, learning and memory and executive function including planning and organisation.

Inflammation and depression are connected. While it is not possible to say that one causes the other, we do know that up to half of people living with autoimmune diseases, chronic inflammatory diseases and chronic pain experience depression and/or anxiety. As is the case with almost every underlying health condition associated with brain fog, women are at increased risk of depression.

Hormones most probably play a role too. Oestrogen promotes brain health and boosts mood. Mental health can decline along with oestrogen levels. Progesterone may exacerbate anxiety and PTSD. People with premenstrual dysphoric disorder (PMDD) experience severe irritability, depression or anxiety in the week or two before their period.

Assessment: Depression*

Once you have filled in the table below, check the scores table underneath to get the values for each of your choices. Enter them in the score column.

Tick the box that best describes how you have felt over the last week. During the past week …	Rarely or none of the time: < 1 day	Some or a little of the time: 1–2 days	Occasionally or a moderate amount of the time: 3–4 days	All of the time: 5–7 days	Score
1. I was bothered by things that don't usually bother me					
2. I did not feel like eating, my appetite was poor					
3. I felt that I could not shake off the blues, even with help from my family					
4. I felt that I was just as good as other people					
5. I had trouble keeping my mind on what I was doing					

*Centre for Epidemiological Studies – Depression (CES-D Scale)

Tick the box that best describes how you have felt over the last week. During the past week ...	Rarely or none of the time: < 1 day	Some or a little of the time: 1–2 days	Occasionally or a moderate amount of the time: 3–4 days	All of the time: 5–7 days	Score
6. I felt depressed					
7. I felt that everything I did was an effort					
8. I felt hopeful about the future					
9. I thought my life had been a failure					
10. I felt fearful					
11. My sleep was restless					
12. I was happy					
13. I talked less than usual					
14. I felt lonely					
15. People were unfriendly					
16. I enjoyed life					
17. I had crying spells					
18. I felt sad					
19. I felt that people disliked me					
20. I could not 'get going'					
Total					

Scores:

Statements	Rarely or none of the time: < 1 day	Some or a little of the time: 1–2 days	Occasionally or a moderate amount of time: 3–4 days	All of the time: 5–7 days
4, 8, 12 and 16	3	2	1	0
All other statements	0	1	2	3

Add all items together to get your total score ___

While a score of sixteen or higher is considered depressed, it is important to note that this is not a diagnostic tool. If you are concerned that you might be depressed, it is important that you seek professional help sooner rather than later.

How does stress work?

Your brain determines what is threatening. It also accumulates pertinent memories about a stressor and regulates your physiological and behavioural responses to it. There are two key systems involved in the stress response: the fast-acting autonomic nervous system and the slower hypothalamic-pituitary-adrenal (HPA) axis which you encountered in Chapter 4 on hormones.

The amygdala (centre of fear and emotions), the hippocampus (critical for learning and memory) and the prefrontal cortex (thinking and decision-making) are also involved and are of particular interest in terms of brain fog symptoms. The stress response leads to the release of adrenaline and cortisol. As adrenaline circulates through your body, it triggers physiological changes that happen so quickly you aren't consciously aware of them.

Your heart beats faster than normal, pumping blood to your muscles. Your sweat glands contract, squeezing sweat droplets onto your skin. Your breathing speeds up so you can take in as much oxygen as possible and your brain receives extra oxygen, increasing alertness. Your sight, hearing and other senses become sharper. Energy-providing glucose (blood sugar) is released into your bloodstream. All of this happens to ensure that you have the best chance of survival.

Your amygdala and your hypothalamus set all of this in motion before your visual system has had a chance to fully process what is happening. Sensory information, for example a loud bang or the roar of an engine, travels to your amygdala via two separate routes: a short pathway and a long pathway. The sensory information is first routed straight to your amygdala (short route) leading to your first, fast, startled reaction. The long pathway allows the same information to be sent to your thinking brain for processing before sending it to the amygdala.

Your thinking brain evaluates the information and assigns meaning to it and determines whether it is really threatening or not, then your amygdala is informed and produces an appropriate response. The long route brings your awareness to the actuality of the situation, allowing you to establish whether you are in danger or whether you have, in fact, been startled by a harmless balloon bursting. The changes happen so quickly that you aren't consciously aware of them but this first, fast, reaction will save your life, getting you to jump back out of the way of an oncoming car without having to think about it. After the threat has passed (the car is gone) or after your thinking brain has determined that there was no actual threat to you (it was a balloon bursting not gunfire), your parasympathetic system takes over and brings your body back to a balanced state.

Within fifteen to twenty minutes of a stressful event, the hormone cortisol is released. Cortisol has become known as the stress hormone but like the other hormones discussed in Chapter 4, it has receptors throughout your body so can trigger lots of different actions, depending on the type of cell that it is acting on. When released as part of the stress response, cortisol mobilises energy to respond to the demands of your behavioural response (e.g. fight or flight) to the stressor by either activating or suppressing different processes in your body. Cortisol may also suppress bodily processes not essential for survival in the moment, including immunity, digestion and growth. The release of cortisol is regulated by a negative feedback mechanism, which means that as cortisol levels rise, they block the further release of the hormone, ultimately leading to a drop in cortisol levels.

The release of the stress hormones cortisol and adrenaline in an acute response enhance muscular activity so that you have the strength to fight or the speed to flee. The flow of these hormones to your hippo-campus helps you to remember those notable moments, supporting your survival in the future. In this way, your memory will remind you not to go down a similar dark alley in the future, or recall how you managed to overcome or escape your attacker. Once the threat has passed, the stress response restores homeostasis via its negative feedback mechanism, cortisol levels return to baseline and your nervous system shifts you from fight or flight mode to rest-and-digest mode.

Chronic stress can disrupt this natural rhythm and also interfere with circadian rhythms and sleep which, as you learned in the previous chapter, when disrupted can result in brain fog symptoms. An ongoing stressor – such as chronic illness, chronic pain, money issues or relationship problems – that last for extended periods can repeatedly elevate the neurophysiological stress response or fail to shut it off when not needed. When this occurs, the same physiological mechanisms that are helpful in an acute situation can upset your body's biochemical balance, disrupting homeostasis, accelerating disease and giving rise to brain fog symptoms including impaired learning and memory.

Remember that the stress response is neither good nor bad; it simply evolved and exists to support your survival, which it does extremely well in acute situations. It just becomes problematic when stress is prolonged or poorly managed.

How does stress contribute to brain fog?

Your prefrontal cortex, your hippocampus and your amygdala are the key players in both the stress response and memory function. Chronic stress impacts on neuroplasticity in all three structures, enhancing it in the amygdala but – and this has particular relevance for brain fog – impairing it in the prefrontal cortex and the hippocampus.

The first studies on the impact of stress on cognitive function came about after it was noticed during the Second World War that pilots who were highly skilled often crashed their planes during the stress of battle due to mental errors. Early research that tried to understand this phenomenon showed that stress impaired performance on tasks that required complex, flexible thinking (which we now know relies on the prefrontal cortex) but improved performance on easier, habitual or well-rehearsed tasks (which rely on the basal ganglia).

Stress is associated with a loss of neural networks in the prefrontal cortex, interfering with executive function. Your prefrontal cortex allows you to make decisions, judge situations and determine appropriate behaviour in social situations. Through neural networks, it also supports working memory, allowing you, for example, to maintain information about an event that has just occurred while you simultaneously access information from your past experience and use the combined information to inform your decisions, regulate your behaviour and thinking, monitor your emotions and modify your emotional behavioural responses. If executive function is one of the domains you identified as affected in your brain fog profile you will know only too well how debilitating it can be if it stops working as it should. As the prefrontal cortex is particularly vulnerable to stress, if chronic or long-term stress is at the root of your brain fog, managing it should alleviate your executive function symptoms, restoring your ability to make decisions, plan and think clearly.

When the amygdala activates stress pathways under conditions of psychological stress it leads to the release of high levels of noradren-aline[24] and dopamine,[25] which impair prefrontal cortex control (rational thinking) but enhance amygdala function (fear). As a consequence, behaviour patterns switch from slow, thoughtful, rational responses to rapid, reflexive, emotional responses. Rather than considering your mum's suggestion about how to improve your baking, you sarcastically snap at her that you're sorry your efforts don't live up to her high standards. While switching the brain from thoughtful, reflective regulation by the prefrontal cortex to more rapid, reflexive regulation by the amygdala might save your life if you actually are in acute danger and need to act fast, it can have negative effects in most other situations when you need to make choices that require thoughtful analysis and the ability to control or inhibit your more impulsive responses.

Flexible thinking is an important skill that allows us to consider different options and adjust our plans when things don't go as expected. It allows us to adopt different perspectives, change our behaviour and adapt to changing circumstances and environments. It also allows us to reframe stressors as challenges. Cognitive flexibility is critical for stress management and coping. This flexibility also prevents us from getting 'stuck' or thinking obsessively about one thing. The relationship between the prefrontal cortex and the hippocampus is particularly important for flexible thinking and for consolidating memories. Chronic stress disrupts this relationship in a way that makes the amygdala's fear response stronger and hinders the ability of the hippocampus to update memories with new information. This results in a shift from flexible cognitive learning to more rigid, habit-like behaviour. Instead of being flexible and adapting to a new situation, we persist with old habits that may no longer be effective or appropriate.

This stress-induced pattern of brain activity can impact on your ability to make choices that promote healthy brain function. Loss of executive control during stress can also lead to relapse of a number of behaviours that impact negatively on brain function. You might find yourself drinking alcohol to excess and overeating, for example. Ex-smokers and people with addiction problems are also more likely to relapse in times of stress. Prolonged stress can also leave you vulnerable to depression.

Chronic stress increases BDNF (Miracle-Gro for the brain) in the amygdala but decreases it in the hippocampus. Essentially, what this means is that chronic stress strengthens the structures in your brain that promote the stress response and weakens the structures that provide negative feedback on the stress response, impairing your ability to control it or switch it off.

Stress-induced structural changes to the hippocampus require several weeks of stress exposure but changes in the prefrontal cortex can begin after just one week of continuous stress. Thankfully, animal research suggests that the changes that occur in the prefrontal cortex and in the hippocampus are reversible, which is a good incentive to start managing stress now. If you have been chronically stressed for some time it means that you will need to work hard to break this negative pattern, but it can be done and the payoff will be worth it.

Our bodies are usually very efficient and, thanks to the negative feedback mechanism, cortisol levels are kept under control. However, when cortisol levels are too high for too long it seems this feedback mechanism gets a little screwed up. Cortisol production may go through the roof or your body may not make enough of it. Or you may make a ton of it at the wrong time when you are trying to sleep and nothing in the morning when you need it to get out of bed.

As discussed in detail in the previous chapter, poor sleep can cause brain fog symptoms. In addition, insufficient sleep at night boosts stress hormones and stress, particularly prolonged or poorly managed stress, which can interfere with sleep. A vicious cycle can ensue where more stress leads to less sleep and less sleep leads to more stress. This is due, in part, to the fact that brain chemicals associated with deep sleep are the same ones that tell your body to stop producing stress hormones. Stress hormones peak in the afternoon and evening making it more difficult to get to sleep. The resulting brain fog, exhaustion, fatigue and irritability make it hard to focus, solve problems and maintain relationships, leading to more stress and so on it goes.

While the relationship between sleep and stress is clear, the degree to which stress impacts on sleep is not the same for everyone. People like me, who experience a drastic deterioration in sleep when exposed to stress, are said to have a highly reactive sleep system. In contrast, people like my husband, with low sleep reactivity, can be exposed to the same amount of stress without any impact on their sleep patterns. The degree to which exposure to stress disrupts your sleep is trait-like and is influenced by your genetic heritage. If you are a woman and/or come from a family with a history of insomnia you are more likely to have a highly reactive sleep system. High sleep reactivity is linked to increased risk for insomniac disorder, shift worker disorder, depression and anxiety – all of which can produce symptoms of brain fog. Even more reason to manage stress.

When you appraise a situation or event as stressful, you allocate cognitive resources to coping. This results in a lower cognitive performance than during non-stressful times – you have less capacity to carry out cognitive tasks like processing information or making a decision. If you are preoccupied with a stressor and find yourself either replaying a past stressful encounter over and over or worrying about some event that might happen at a point in the future, it impacts on your cognitive functioning in the here and now.

In these circumstances, short-term stress impacts on your cognitive functioning by reducing your ability to pay attention, keep track of what you are doing or saying or your capacity to remember steps in a task at hand. We all have our moments, but when they become a regular part of your life, such as frequently going blank mid-sentence, it can become downright scary. These kinds of symptoms can also cause you to withdraw from social situations and make other decisions that affect the quality of your life for fear of embarrassment.

Short-term stress is associated with short-term increases in inflammation and negative mood, both of which are associated with fatigue, which might explain reductions in your capacity to pay attention. Chronic stress in the long term is consistently associated with poorer cognitive performance. It increases biological wear and tear, hormones get messed up, inflammation is increased and the neural structures that underlie cognitive function undergo stress-induced changes, so it's no wonder your brain feels foggy.

Practical tips to manage stress

If you are chronically stressed it may feel that there is nothing you can do about it, but you have a lot more control than you might think. Understanding your attitude to stress, the way you think, the stories that you tell yourself about stress and your perceptions of stress will help you to find ways to break the hold that stress has on your life and start clearing the fog.

Aiming for a more balanced life with time for work, leisure and relationships is key. You may be thinking, 'How can I make time for leisure and relationships when I already feel overwhelmed with work and looking after the kids?' but you have the power to make different choices when it comes to your responses, thoughts and actions. Building balance into your life and gaining an understanding of your own beliefs, attitudes and responses to stress will help you to build resilience to challenges and better manage stress on an ongoing basis. Experiment with the stress-management tips below till you find what works best for you.

1. Choose your thoughts carefully

When it comes to stress what you think really matters. Thinking about a stressor can activate the physiological stress response, releasing adrenaline and cortisol. If you constantly think stressful or negative thoughts or obsess about what can go wrong, your body will continue responding as if you are under threat. Eventually, a finely tuned response designed to save your life in an acute situation becomes a constant state taking a terrible toll on your body and your brain in the process.

The stress response evolved to give you the strength to fight off an assailant or run as fast as you have ever run in your life to escape. You do not need this kind of energy to deal with a thought, especially a thought that you probably don't need to have in the first place. Far better to take control of your thinking, adapt your attitude and introduce practical measures to manage stress and your response to it on an ongoing basis.

As a first step, you need to identify the sources of stress in your life. Acute and major stressors like bereavement, money and relationship issues are relatively easy to identify. If you have completed the stress log in this chapter you will have a good idea of what in your life could be contributing to your chronic stress and brain fog.

We have a tendency to look outward for sources of stress, overlooking how much our own thoughts, beliefs, behaviours and feelings contribute to everyday stress levels. For example, maybe you are constantly stressed by the fact that you need to work late and long hours to get projects completed – could it be your unnecessary perfectionism that is driving the longer working hours rather than the actual work demands?

Revisit your stress log and take a closer look at your habits, attitude and the stories that you tell to explain stress to yourself and to others. Do you say stress is just part and parcel of your job, your relationship or your home life? Do you say things like 'It's the nature of the job' or 'It's always mad around here' or 'I'm just that sort of person, I've a lot of nervous energy'? Perhaps you say stress is temporary or transitory – 'Oh things are just crazy right now' – when the reality is that things in your life are always crazy. Have you come to view chronic stress as entirely normal and unexceptional? Or perhaps you take no responsibility for the stress in your life and blame it on other people or things that 'happen' to you.

To gain this control and end chronic stress you need to identify and accept responsibility for the role that you play in making and maintaining it. It might take some time to tease this apart. In addition to completing the stress log you might find it useful to keep a stress journal on an ongoing basis. As well as enabling you to see patterns and common themes, it may help you keep yourself on track if old habits and stressful thinking start to creep back in. In addition to the items you noted for your stress log, you could record how you felt emotionally, physically and cognitively at the time and what you did to feel better.

If you believe that the events in your life are controlled by outside forces then you have what's referred to as an external locus of control.

In contrast, if you believe that you are the master of your own destiny you have what's referred to as an internal locus of control. What you believe about your ability to control important aspects of your life will shape your attitude.

Are you someone who tends to see events as passively happening to you, determined by luck, fate or chance? Or are you someone who feels in control of your own destiny, playing a very active role in your successes and failures and in shaping your life? People who feel they play an active role in shaping their lives tend to be happier, less stressed and less depressed than people who place control outside themselves. Anxiety is closely linked to our perception of control so people who abdicate control to others and to external forces are more prone to anxiety.

2. Practice acceptance

Acceptance is not passive or weak. Acceptance is an active response that requires strength and promotes resilience. Where the source of stress such as losing a loved one is unavoidable, accepting their passing rather than railing against their death represents the least stressful approach and is the most beneficial to your health. Globally stressful events, like an economic downturn, a pandemic or a natural disaster, are beyond your control so there is no point in stressing out over them. Fighting or fleeing are not options. Far better to focus on things that you can control such as how you react to the stressor and what practical steps you can take to adapt and survive.

Acceptance and forgiveness are closely linked. I doubt that holding grudges and withholding forgiveness offer any positive health benefits but accepting the fact that the world is not perfect and the reality that people make mistakes will free you of unnecessary stress and negative energy. Let go of any anger and resentment that you are holding on to. No grand gestures are required; you don't have to forgive someone face to face (though you can of course if you wish), all you need to do to manage your stress is release the resentful, angry thoughts that stress you and move on.

When you have to deal with a stressor that you can't change, remember that you can change yourself. Altering your expectations and attitude can give you back a sense of control. Never lose sight of the big picture. How important is the stressor that you are currently facing in the grand scheme of things? Living through COVID-19 helped many of us to adjust our perspectives. Many things that pre-pandemic we were chronically stressed about became inconsequential.

If you feel stress rising, ask yourself as early as possible, 'How important is this, will it matter next month, next year, is it worth getting upset for?' If the answer is no, then let it go and focus your energy elsewhere on something that does matter. Reframing stressors can help. Instead of seeing being stuck in a traffic jam as a stressful waste of time, reframe it as your downtime, time to listen to a podcast, audiobook or find a good radio station.

3. Look for silver linings

Look for silver linings. When you experience a major stressor, like being made redundant, try to view it as an opportunity. While that sounds like a platitude, it doesn't take away from the truth of the statement. I can testify to that from personal experience. As I write this, we are in the midst of the COVID-19 pandemic. Because my research involves face-to-face contact it cannot currently continue and so this week my research team and I were let go by the university. This was stressful not because I have been let go but because my team have been made redundant. Hopefully by the time this book is published we will be able to resume our research and reemploy the team. Who knows when I will be able to give talks again or when I will be able to travel? But there is always a silver lining – in this case, not working at the university and enforced self-isolation mean that I have more time to devote to writing this book and to recording my 'Super Brain' podcast. There is no point in getting stressed over what is gone; I am focused in the moment and trust that my brain will come up with a post-pandemic plan that allows me to continue my mission within the constraints of the new normal.

A simple shift in perspective can make a huge difference when it comes to choosing your thoughts and managing your stress. Close your eyes for a moment and imagine the feeling that you get in your gut when you feel stressed, anxious or nervous. Stay with it and take note of what it feels like and where you feel it. Now open your eyes and erase that feeling.

Take a breath.

Now close your eyes again and imagine the feeling that you get in your gut when you feel excited, when you are anticipating something good that is about to happen. Think of the butterflies you feel in your tummy when you catch eyes with someone you really fancy. Stay with it and take note of what it feels like.

Now open your eyes and consciously compare the feelings of stress and excitement.

The truth of the matter is that the only difference between these feelings is that you name one 'stress' and the other 'excitement'. But each of those words come with a cascade of feelings, physiological changes and health consequences, positive and negative depending on the name. This is, I think, a great illustration of the power of thinking and how we perceive events and feelings. Next time you get that wobbly feeling in your gut, try naming it as excitement rather than stress. The feelings are practically identical, so it's your choice.

Stress is a natural part of living. It keeps us motivated and allows us to adapt to change and to become more resilient. Life would be boring and static without challenge, uncertainty and novelty. What would your life be like if you never went on that first date, attended that job interview or made that speech? If you manage your stress and stressors well by preparing properly and seeking support when needed, stressful events can be an opportunity for personal growth and achievement. You will still feel the fear and often want to flee, but when you come out the other side you reap the rewards and will feel invigorated, alive and proud. Don't forget to look back on those moments in life where you felt the fear and did it anyway, where you reaped the rewards of bravery – those memories may spur you on today. A small shift in perspective from fear to excitement can make a huge difference. Remember, courage grows out of fear.

My favourite stress busters are smiling and laughter. Laughing with other people is rewarding, it boosts bonding and reduces stress and anxiety. Although the neural basis of laughter is not well understood, it is thought to act a bit like an antidepressant, raising serotonin levels in the brain and elevating your mood. When your brain is overloaded with information it looks for biofeedback from your body. By smiling you can send signals to your brain to trigger the release of brain chemicals that can help to dissipate stress and anxiety. Don't be afraid to laugh at yourself. Stressed individuals with a strong sense of humour become less depressed and anxious than stressed individuals with a less well-developed sense of humour.

Negative thinking can be both a source and a consequence of stress and is a common symptom of anxiety. Practising positive thinking not only helps reduce stress but also has very real brain-health benefits. Try writing down your negative thoughts. The simple act of putting them on paper may release your brain from having to remember them. Humans have a natural propensity to notice the negative, so reframing your thoughts to be positive instead does take a bit of work. For every negative thought you have, make a conscious effort to have five positive thoughts to counteract the negative effect.

4. Be practical

Be realistic about what you can achieve. Recognise when good enough is better than perfect. Also, be realistic about what those around you, such as work colleagues, employees, friends and family, can achieve. If your husband always forgets stuff at the shops or buys the wrong brand you can either accept this and laugh about it as we do in my family or you can take practical steps to change it. For example, by texting more explicit lists or sending photos of the exact brand so your husband has a visual reference to guide him in the shop. If that fails, perhaps you could do the shopping and delegate a different task that your husband can excel at.

If a friend repeatedly disappoints you by failing to show up for events that are important to you, causing you stress before, after and during the event, ask yourself why you keep asking her to attend. Her past behaviour will predict her future behaviour, so it is likely that the pattern will continue to repeat unless you break it by inviting someone more reliable or attending the events on your own. You might be surprised how enjoyable the events become when you are not anxiously watching the door for her arrival. If you want to minimise your stress you need to either accept the other person's behaviour, adjust your own behaviour or modify your expectations. You have control over these options. The choice is yours.

Striving for perfection is a recipe for stress; it is rarely attainable and you may well find that what you produce within normal working hours already exceeds the expectations of others. I am happy to say that I am a reformed perfectionist. As a child, I believed that anything less than full marks was failure. I believed that perfectionism was a positive ideal. But I was wrong – perfectionism is a major source of avoidable stress. Perfectionists set themselves up for failure in every single thing that they do. Perfection is unattainable so you will always fall short. Far, far better to set reasonable standards and learn to be happy with 'good enough' from yourself and others rather than endure the endless disappointment of falling short of perfect. To be honest, 'good enough' for a perfectionist is usually a damn high standard.

Learn to manage your time more effectively. This can take a while to figure out but can really help to eliminate unnecessary stress. It's worth identifying adjustments that you can make to help you use your time better. This will also help you to learn your limits and set boundaries in all areas of your life. You must learn to say no to requests when you simply don't have the time or because carrying out the activity itself would create unwelcome stress rather than add value. Know your limits and stick to them. Taking on more than you can handle is a recipe for stress. Getting to know your motivations for saying yes will help to distinguish between should, must, need and 'want to' activities. Overstretching yourself can lead you to focus only on the things that stress you to the exclusion of other activities in your life, like hobbies, exercise and socialising, which would help you to keep stress in check.

Calendars tend to have hour-long slots and so we often book meetings back-to-back, failing to allow time in between for bathroom breaks, a breather or even just time to switch gear and refresh from one meeting to the next. There is no reason that every meeting needs to begin on the hour – live a little and schedule some for 10 past or 10 to the hour to give yourself some me time and some pee time.

Prioritise tasks, break projects down into manageable actions and delegate responsibility when you can. Prune your to-do list by dropping tasks that are neither important nor urgent. Adapt or change your environment. It is possible for you to exert control over some factors in your external environment. If the news or someone's posts on social media are stressing you out, mute them, turn off the TV or radio, switch off news alerts on your phone and log off social media. You'll gain some precious time for less stressful activities too. If traffic stresses you out consider an alternative means of transport, an alternative route or travel time.

Your body likes regularity and needs internal balance to maintain health. Stress can disrupt this balance in a way that can have serious consequences for health. Eat and exercise regularly. Eating balanced nutritious meals throughout the day will help to clear your head and give your brain the energy it needs to get you through stressful times. Reducing the amount of caffeine and sugar you consume will help to make you feel more relaxed. Go to bed at a regular hour each day and allow your body time to rest and recuperate after stressful events. Set boundaries to ensure you have a good balance between work and the rest of your life. Make sure that you have time for social activities, family life, responsibilities, solitary pursuits and relaxation. Switch off email notifications and only check your messages at pre-determined times.

If you can, treat work as a place, not a thing. For my first full-time job, I worked in a large life assurance company with offices in the city centre. There were no mobile phones, no email and no one worked from home. Work was something that I did when I was physically in the office. I wasn't contactable outside of the physical space of that office. In fact, no one would have dreamt of breaching the boundary between work and the rest of your life. All of that has changed dramatically. It is the rare individual who doesn't feel constantly 'on' and always 'contactable'. Modern technology has no respect for boundaries. While I appreciate the benefits of accessibility and remote working, there is a lot to be said for the days when the physical walls of your workplace acted as a boundary within which your work remained. Roll back the years if you can and constrain work to a specific place and time. You can minimise stress by only dealing with work emails and phone calls when you are in that place during designated working hours.

Make time for hobbies, socialising and relaxing. Sometimes stress fools us into putting the blinkers on and forgetting to do things that interest us. Hobbies can seem unimportant and even a frivolous waste of time when we have so much to do. But engaging with hobbies that interest us is a wonderful stress buster that can give a real sense of achievement when feeling under-stimulated and simultaneously over-whelmed by other aspects of life. Hobbies can challenge your brain and provide opportunities for learning and fun by allowing you to make use of some of your best skills. They have the capacity to totally engage you to the point where you lose track of time and find distance from the stressors in your life.

Carve out some 'me time'. Nurture yourself, make time for fun and relaxation. Don't allow work, responsibilities or obligations to encroach on this time. You need to recharge your batteries away from all demands. Make sure that you do at least one thing that you enjoy every day. It can be something simple like lighting a scented candle and letting the aroma relax you.

Consider learning relaxation techniques such as yoga, deep breathing and meditation. You could also try self-massage using aromatherapy oils or even just a simple moisturiser. Apply the oil or moisturiser slowly using your fingers and thumbs to massage the muscles as you work the cream or oil into your skin. Spend extra time on the soles of your feet, calves, thighs and arms and don't forget to massage your hands. Place one arm, palm up, on your thigh. Starting at your upper arm, using the heel of your other hand push slowly down towards your wrist with enough pressure to feel some heat. Do the same over the mound of your thumb and down your palm towards your fingertips. Repeat several times, then swap hands. For your back, consider using a foam roller or even a tennis ball positioned between your back and the floor. Gently move your body up and down and from side to side focusing on areas where the muscles feel tight. A foam roller will work well for your thighs too.

One of my favourite things is when my hairdresser gives me a head massage at the basin. It's just so relaxing I could stay there all day. I've recently learned how to give myself a head massage and whilst it's never going to be the same as getting a proper head massage, it's still incredibly relaxing. Here's how: using your fingertips massage your scalp as if you were washing your hair for a couple of minutes. Draw little circles along your hairline, above your eyebrows and along your cheeks. Place the heel of your hand on either side of your head along your temples under your hair. Push your scalp upwards, hold for a couple of seconds and release. Work your way around your scalp repeating this movement. Take your hair in sections and pull away from the scalp. Enjoy!

Have a strategy to relieve stress in the moment. Take a deep breath and use your senses or a soothing movement. It may take a bit of experimenting to find something that works specifically for you. Inhaling an aromatherapy scent or lighting an aromatherapy candle works wonders for me. For you it might be the taste of peppermint gum, music, a photograph, visualising a relaxing place, snuggling with your dog. Don't rely on alcohol, drugs, unhealthy eating or compulsive behaviours to reduce stress – ultimately they will make you, and those around you, more rather than less stressed.

Going for a run, dancing or doing sit-ups can also work as excellent stress busters. Exercise and all sorts of physical activity reduce stress and release endorphins that make you feel good. Exercise also improves mental health, reducing levels of anxiety. Spending most of the day sitting without moving can increase anxiety levels, so make time to move around. Even five minutes of aerobic exercise can stimulate anti-anxiety effects.

5. Be in the moment

When we are stressed, it can be difficult to keep focused on the task at hand. Being present and focused on what you are doing while you are doing it is a natural antidote to stress-induced absentmindedness. Being 'in the moment' also helps you to stay away from negative thoughts or memories that can cause anxiety, stress and depression. Rooting awareness in your body by, for example, feeling the soles of your feet connect with the ground while you walk or by focusing on breathing in and out, can tie you closer to the present moment.

6. Be connected

Resist the temptation to socially withdraw when stressed. Seek support from friends, family and, if necessary, health professionals. Choose wisely who you spend time with when you are stressed. You need support, not someone who will add to your stress. If someone consistently causes stress in your life, consider limiting the amount of time you spend with them or step away from the relationship altogether.

Talk to someone you trust. Sharing what you are going through can be incredibly helpful. Sometimes just saying something out loud can make you realise how you have blown it out of proportion or may help you to realise that you have completely misread a situation. Even, or especially, when there is nothing that you or anyone can do about a stressor, talking to someone can be cathartic. We need other people to make us feel safe. Volunteering for an organisation that helps others can be a fantastic way to put your troubles in perspective. The opportunity to focus your attention on others and away from yourself can act as a form of stress relief in and of itself.

Communicate what you are feeling sooner rather than later. Don't let things build up to the point that they explode at an inappropriate time in an unhelpful way. If something is bothering you at work, communicate it as soon as possible in a factual, respectful, assertive way. Seek solutions rather than let resentment build. Be willing to come to a compromise; finding a middle ground may be enough to relieve your stress.

Face-to-face interactions with other people can trigger the release of hormones that counteract the physiological stress response. Make sure you connect regularly in person with a network of people you trust to have your best interests at heart. Don't worry about being a burden; most people are happy, even flattered that you would confide in them. Don't forget to return the favour, everyone needs a good listener. You don't have to be able to solve their problems or take on their stressors, just let them offload to you. Listening to others can also give you a fresh take on your own stress and help you to find solutions. If your stressor or the nature of your friends and family means that there is no one you can trust to offload to, consider talking to your GP or a therapist trained in stress-management techniques.

Key chapter takeaways

- Forgetfulness, loss of sense of humour, poor sleep, unhealthy eating and feelings of loneliness are signs of stress.
- The stress response allows you to respond to a stressor and return your body to optimal conditions.
- Psychological stress refers to the extent to which a person perceives that their demands exceed their ability to cope.
- Prolonged or poorly managed chronic stress can negatively impact on your health, affecting your behaviour and your brain function.
- Well-managed stress will help you to adapt to your environment and make you more resilient.
- Chronic stress can interfere with circadian rhythms and sleep.
- Repeated elevation of the stress response can upset your body's biochemical balance and give rise to brain fog and multiple other health issues.
- With chronic stress, behaviour patterns switch from slow, thoughtful responses to rapid, reflexive, emotional responses.
- Stress impairs cognitive function because the resources ordinarily available to the cognitive task are taken up by thinking or worrying about the stressor.
- Changing your thinking, perceptions and attitudes can help you to better manage stress.
- Acceptance is a valid, active and appropriate response to stressors beyond your control.
- Smiling and laughter are natural stress busters.
- Striving for perfection is a recipe for ongoing stress.
- Accept good enough and be realistic about what you and others can achieve.
- Aim for balance across all aspects of your life: exercise, diet, sleep, work, leisure, relaxation.
- Resist the temptation to socially withdraw when stressed; instead reach out to family and friends for support.
- If necessary seek professional help from a GP or therapist trained

in stress-management techniques.

Get ready for the 30-day plan

Gather together the following items before you start the 30-day plan:

1. Create a sensory box containing:

    a. Something that you love the smell of
    b. Something that you love the feel of
    c. Something that you like to look at
    d. Something that you like the taste of
    e. Something that you like the sound of

Place the items in a box, container or drawer in your bedroom or bathroom or somewhere you can access them easily first thing every morning.

2. Buy a notebook

Place it together with a pen or pencil beside your bed. It can be a simple copybook or a really fancy journal. The point is to have somewhere that you can write. I personally like to choose a notebook with a pretty or tactile cover because I find that I want to pick it up to experience its texture and enjoy how it looks.

Change: Exercise

Are you getting enough?

When was the last time you tried something new? I'm not talking new clothes or new shoes here. Seriously, when was the last time you consciously made an effort to exercise your brain? You need to stimulate your brain to promote the growth of new brain cells and the connections between them.

What about your body? Are you getting onough physical exercise? Maybe you've stopped exercising because you feel mentally fatigued? Bad move, because physical inactivity can contribute to brain fog. No matter how tired you feel, if you want to beat brain fog you'll need to get moving. The more steps (literally) you take to get fitter, the healthier your brain becomes.

Ernestine Shepherd is an eighty-four-year-old body builder and competitive runner. In 2010, at the age of seventy-four, she was declared the oldest competitive body builder in the world by *Guinness World Records*. But at fifty-six, Ernestine Shepherd was a 'well-padded' 'slug' (I'm quoting from her website) who had never worked out a day in her life. One day, while she and her sister were shopping for swimsuits, the ladies laughed at themselves in the mirror and made a pact to join a gym together to get into better shape. Alas, a short time later

Ernestine's sister died suddenly. Devasted, Ernestine stopped going to the gym. A few months later, a friend suggested that the grieving Ernestine return to the gym to finish what she started with her sister Velvet (what a great name). The rest, as they say, is history.

If you google Ernestine, you will see incredible images of a woman in her eighties with sculpted muscles and an incredibly well-defined six-pack. Starting slowly in her fifties under the guidance of an expert trainer, she transformed not only her body but her life too. Ernestine, who has enjoyed life-changing success since committing to exercise, also says that she has never been happier. She has more energy than ever before despite running ten miles a day and doing strength training four days a week.

Extensive research shows that engaging in aerobic exercise (e.g. running, dancing, swimming laps, cycling, etc.) benefits your brain and improves various cognitive functions including those commonly affected in brain fog. Research also indicates that regularly engaging in both aerobic exercise and resistance training, as Ernestine does, improves cognitive function in adults over fifty.

Put down this book for a second and curl your biceps. It's just muscle movement, right? Wrong. Of course flexing your biceps, like any movement, involves your muscles but your central nervous system is also involved in what is actually a complex neuro-muscular process. When you followed my instruction to flex your biceps, electrical signals travelled at warp speed from your brain to your spinal cord and on to your muscles. Any plan to move, whether it's flicking your hair or flexing your biceps, starts in your brain.

Specialised cells in your central nervous system called motor neurons are involved in the movements that you make. Your brain sends an electrical signal to your spinal cord using upper motor neurons. The signal is then passed to lower motor neurons along communication cables that stretch from your spinal cord to your skeletal muscles (e.g. legs, arms, fingers, toes, etc.) where they make contact with the muscle fibres directly. Muscle fibres are actually muscle cells and are incredibly large. When the electrical signal arrives at the muscle fibre, the motor neuron releases a burst of chemicals that trigger the muscle fibre to contract and – hey presto – your bicep is flexed.

When Ernestine repeatedly engages in resistance training (e.g. lifting weights), the cells in her muscles and central nervous system adapt in ways that increase the size and strength of her muscles. Scientists don't know the exact mechanisms but they know that in response to the repeated stress of exercise the cells in the activated muscle grow and the motor neurons recruit more muscle cells, simultaneously producing a synchronous activation of the muscle fibres which helps to strengthen the muscle being trained. This is very different to what happens when you ordinarily move a muscle that you haven't been training. When an untrained muscle is moved, the cells in the muscle fibre are activated in turn. Because of this sequential rather than synchronised activation, untrained muscles have less strength than trained muscles.

Exercise doesn't just strengthen your muscles – other systems and organs, including your brain, benefit too. If you are living with brain fog, particularly if fatigue is one of your symptoms, you might be thinking that exercise is just too challenging, too much like hard work. You are absolutely right, exercise is hard work; it is incredibly challenging but that's the point, that is exactly why it is so beneficial. When you run, walk or engage in any form of physical activity your muscles demand more oxygen. To meet this demand, your lungs and heart have to work harder but, as a consequence of repeatedly rising to the challenge, they eventually become stronger. For example, over time your cardio-vascular system responds to increasing muscle demands by increasing the size of your heart and growing new blood vessels. As your physical fitness improves, your body becomes more efficient at getting oxygen into your bloodstream and transporting it to the working muscles which also increase in size.

Your brain also benefits from a healthy, efficient, cardiovascular system because it can capitalise on a constant, efficient and reliable supply of oxygen and nutrients to optimise functioning. Physical exercise also increases the rate at which new neurons are created in the brain, which is good news because when it comes to brain cells more is better.

Mental exercise is important too because it helps determine how those new neurons are used and how they survive. Regularly lifting weights challenges your muscles and puts them under stress, causing them to adapt and become stronger. The same principle applies to your brain: if you want it to adapt and become stronger you need to challenge it regularly. Challenging your muscles by regularly lifting weights strengthens muscle fibres and other connective tissue in the muscles. Similarly challenging your brain by regularly exercising it will strengthen the connective tissue between brain cells, helping them to function better and faster. This neuroplasticity, the brain's ability to adapt in response to challenge and change, is an amazing phenomenon. It allows the brain to expand its capacity and will help you to overcome your brain fog and think faster, sharper, better.

You can change your brain

Neuroplasticity is critical for learning and memory.

It takes three to four years to acquire 'the Knowledge' to qualify as a licensed London taxi driver. Knowing the layout of 25,000 streets and the quickest route from A to B is a fantastic feat of learning that illustrates the human capacity to acquire and use knowledge of a large complex city to navigate within it. In 2000, Irish psychologist Eleanor Maguire began a series of intriguing studies investigating the hippo-campal structures in the brains of licensed London taxi drivers. Among other things, your hippocampus facilitates spatial memory, allowing you to navigate your world with ease, whether it's driving the kids to school, walking to work, finding the right lecture theatre, or remembering the quickest route to the airport to catch your flight on time.

The hippocampi in birds whose survival depends on remembering where they stored food are rather large in comparison to the overall size of their brain. In some species, the hippocampi actually enlarge seasonally when there is greater demand on the bird's spatial memory (i.e. how often they have to remember where they found or stored food).

Maguire's first study showed that grey matter density in the hippo-campi in London taxi drivers was larger than in non-taxi-driving controls. Since grey matter is made up of the brain cells and white matter the connections between them, you could say that more brain cells were packed into the taxi drivers' hippocampi compared to non-taxi drivers. They also found that size increased in line with years of navigation experience. Maguire speculated that these differences could come from using and updating spatial representations of the London streets. However, there was no way that Maguire could rule out that driving experience, stress and the possibility of pre-existing anatomical differences could have caused the difference.

She and her team then carried out a series of studies comparing qualified taxi drivers with London bus drivers. She also followed trainee taxi drivers over time. Her team scanned the brains of the bus drivers who navigate London along pre-determined routes and found that the grey matter density in their hippocampi was no different to non-bus driver controls. They then compared the bus drivers and the taxi drivers who were matched for driving experience and levels of stress. The taxi drivers had more grey matter in the back of their hippocampi than the bus drivers, suggesting that spatial knowledge rather than stress or driving experience was actually the reason for this difference.

Maguire's team also carried out a study where they assessed the brains and memory of trainees before and after their four-year training. To acquire their license, trainees have to sit a serious of strict exams to demonstrate their spatial memory of the streets and landmarks within a six-mile radius of Charing Cross Station in London. Maguire found that the taxi drivers who qualified experienced a selective increase in grey matter in the back part of their hippocampi. Their memory profile also changed. Whereas trainees who failed to qualify and control participants showed no structural brain changes. This study of average-IQ adults operating in the real world demonstrates that learning can shape your brain, like exercise shapes your muscles.

The founding father of neuroscience, Santiago Ramón y Cajal, said: 'We could say the cerebral cortex is like a garden planted with innumerable trees – the pyramidal cells – which, thanks to intelligent cultivation, can multiply their branches and sink their roots deeper, producing fruits and flowers of ever greater variety and quality.' Think of your brain as a large forest populated with 86 billion neuronal trees. While each neuronal tree has the same basic structure – a cell body (mission control), dendrites (receivers) and axons (communication cables) – the neurons, like trees, come in many varieties.

There are an estimated 16,000 species of trees in the Amazon, the world's largest rainforest, which covers 40 per cent of South America with 390 billion trees. To date, hundreds of different types of neurons have been identified. Just as trees bend in the wind and lean towards the sun, the human brain adapts to the external environment right across its lifespan. While the rate of change in the brain does decline with age, it doesn't cease and new neurons can manifest until we draw our last breath.

Your brain even has its own fertiliser, brain derived neurotropic factor (BDNF), which I referred to as 'Miracle-Gro' for the brain in earlier chapters. BDNF improves neuronal function, protects cells from stress and cell death and encourages neurons to grow, just as fertiliser encourages plants to grow. BDNF is vital for learning and the good news is that aerobic exercise is associated with increased BDNF concentration and enhanced cognitive function.

How does your brain garden grow?

In 1949, Canadian psychologist Donald Hebb observed that neurons in close proximity to each other tend to be active together in a cohesive synchronistic way, as a unified network. A bit like trained muscle fibres that act in synchrony. He hypothesised that this collective action would ultimately lead to a lasting, enhanced communication between the neurons in the network: 'When an axon of cell A is near enough to excite cell B or consistently takes part in firing it, some growth or metabolic change takes place in one or both cells such that A's efficiency, as one of the cell's firing B, is increased.'

This means that when brain cells communicate frequently with each other, the connection between them strengthens and becomes more efficient. When signals travel the same neural pathway over and over again, their efficiency improves and the speed at which they transmit information increases. Something similar happens when athletes en-gage in regular strength training – signals from the brain are sent to the muscle repeatedly and a pathway is formed. Once this happens, the athlete's technique becomes ingrained, movement becomes more automatic and the athlete won't need to concentrate intensely even if they initially found the movement very challenging.

Profit by new experience

During the 1940s, Donald Hebb took some of his lab rats home for his children to play with as pets. Weird I know, but that's a discussion for another book. Several weeks later, when assessing their performance on problem-solving tests (the rats, not his children), he noticed that the 'pet rats' outperformed the 'lab rats'. He interpreted this to mean that early, enriched experience can have a dramatic and permanent effect on brain development and function – he said: 'The richer experience of the pet group . . . made them better able to profit by new experience at maturity.'

Even though Hebb was ahead of his time when he proposed the idea that memories are formed when synaptic connections are strengthened, he wasn't the first to put the idea out there. In 1780, naturalist Charles Bonnet and anatomist Michele Vincenzo Malacarne tested the idea that mental exercise can induce brain growth by taking pairs of dogs and birds and training one from each pair. At post mortem, the trained animals had more folds in their cerebella (the tennis ball bit at the back of the brain) than the untrained animals. The cerebellum plays a key role in learning motor tasks, adapting and fine-tuning to make more accurate movements through trial and error, such as a dog might do when learning to catch a frisbee on the volley or as you might do when learning to hit a baseball, return a serve in tennis, kick a football, catch a rugby ball or shoot a basketball through the hoop or indeed learn ballet, ballroom or street dance.

When the brains of healthy controls are compared with the brains of karate black belts, the experts, who after years of training are able to perform rapid, complex movements, have significantly more communication cables (white matter tracts) in their cerebella and in their motor cortex than the controls. Because this kind of study only compares the brains of the two groups at a single point in time, it is not possible to say categorically that these differences were directly due to their karate training. It could simply be that the expert individuals were born with brains that predisposed them to acquiring the motor skills more easily than others. Studies that scanned the expert and control brains over time would be needed to determine whether the differences observed in the karate experts were actually due to training. Studies that followed people over time as they learned to juggle have shown that it leads to an increased number of brain cells (grey matter density) in an area of the brain that contains motion sensor neurons and to an increased number of communication cables (white matter tracts) in an area of the brain critical for coordinating arm and eye movements.

Amazing as neuroplasticity is, it can sometimes be maladaptive. Prolonged pain of the type discussed in Chapter 5 can give rise to reorganisation of the circuits involved in processing and transmitting painful stimuli to the brain. These changes can persist long after the original cause of the pain, leading to chronic pain and associated brain fog. Addictive, recreational and prescription drugs can hijack brain systems involved in reward, motivation, habit formation, fear, anxiety and emotion, leading to cravings, compulsions and drug-seeking behaviour.

To recap, in order to harness neuroplasticity to help you to beat brain fog you need to a) challenge your brain regularly and b) experience new things.

Exercising your brain

Experiencing new things, meeting new people and encountering new situations is a great way to harness your brain's neuroplasticity and enrich the connections between your brain cells. You don't have to do anything dramatic; your brain will benefit once there is novelty involved. Make a conscious effort to seek out 'first times' in multiple areas of your life. It can be something really simple like listening to a genre of music that you have never listened to before. The opportunities are endless. Let your imagination run amok. Read a book from an unfamiliar genre or read a different section of the newspaper. Tune in to a different radio station than the one you regularly listen to. Take time to read about cultures or viewpoints that are novel to you. Try a new restaurant or order something different from the menu in your favourite restaurant, preferably something you've never tasted before. Try walking a new route to work. Change your jogging route. Take up a new sport, try a new craft or learn a new technique for your favourite hobbies or artistic pursuits. Visit new places, find opportunities to meet new people, become a tourist in your own city.

It is critical to remember that the neurons in your brain need to be challenged in order to reorganise themselves effectively. When you engage in mentally challenging activities it stimulates the connections between brain cells, essentially promoting neuroplasticity. Routine activities don't challenge your brain; you need to push yourself to the next level, try something different or learn something new. The first time you do a crossword it involves learning, which brings brain benefits. Once you are doing crosswords every night it becomes routine so the benefit is very limited. You will need to up the ante to promote neuroplasticity. You could do this, for example, by trying a harder crossword or by setting a time limit within which to solve the crossword. You will need to stretch yourself, push yourself beyond your comfort zone or current ability to induce neuroplasticity and build a stronger more efficient brain. Challenge can be as simple as taking your hobby to the next level, cooking or baking more complicated recipes, learning a new carpentry skill, adding new songs to your repertoire or moving from quick crosswords to cryptic.

Challenging your brain will also impact positively on your mood. Dopamine neurons in your brain become activated when something good happens unexpectedly. The satisfaction that you experience from mastering a challenge like baking a fancy cake, staying upright on a surfboard, playing a new tune or passing your driving test will lead to the release of dopamine, making you feel good, more positive and less depressed. When choosing a challenge, base it on your current abilities, not what you used to be able to do before brain fog. Push yourself just beyond your comfort zone. Your goal needs to be realistic and attainable. Don't go shooting for the stars, stay grounded; there is no reason you can't reach the stars, you just need to make the journey one step at a time.

Dopamine is released when you expect or receive a reward such as food or music, or when you surmount a challenge. Dopamine also tells your brain that whatever you experienced is worth getting more of and so can help you to change your behaviours in ways that will allow you to attain more rewarding experiences and achieve your goals.

The goal of artificial intelligence (AI) is to produce systems that can function intelligently and independently like the human brain. The brain uses its network of neurons to learn things. As you know, we humans can remember the past. We use the data from our past experiences to make models of the world so that we can make predictions. The brain makes inferences about the current state of the world by combining data from our past learning with the incoming signals from our senses which gives the brain new data about the world around us. This allows us to function in the world without, for example, crashing into the furniture in our office.

If the incoming data from our senses doesn't match our internal model created from our past experiences, the brain's prediction will be incorrect. This error drives new learning as the brain has to update its internal model with the new sensory data so that we can navigate the world efficiently and safely. If someone moves the office furniture so that you can no longer use your former route from your desk to the water cooler, your brain learns and updates its internal model by identifying patterns and through trial and error. The more information your brain has about your environment, the better it will be able to compare experiences and predict the probability of certain outcomes. This is why novelty is so important – every new experience you have provides your brain with more data to update the internal model and make more accurate predictions about the world.

By taking advantage of the predictable structure of sensory information, your brain needs to devote fewer attentional resources to the parts that it can predict. This predictive approach frees your brain from having to process and remember every last bit of visual or auditory information it encounters in every moment. It is an efficient use of the brain's limited resources that serves us well. Think back to when you first learned how to drive a car. It took all your energy to remember all of the things that you had to do plus process all of the incoming sensory information at once (e.g. other cars, people, traffic lights, road signs, road marking etc.). Was it terrifying? I remember my palms sweating profusely. Each time you drove the car, each time you made a mistake, you provided your brain with valuable data to update its model of driving and make more accurate predictions which, over time, translated into smooth, safe driving. Before long, you could drive to your destination in one piece without feeling cognitively exhausted. The more driving experience you have and the greater variety of road and weather conditions you encounter, the more accurate your brain's predictions and the better the driver you become.

Paradoxically, the need for predictability drives your brain to seek novelty. Your reward system is most responsive to novelty and unpredictability as this enhances your brain's internal model. Being rewarded by novel events better positions your brain to gain insight from your environment. Novelty also causes your brain to release noradrenaline, which helps to form new brain connections.

Learning is like a powerful brain-changing drug generating new brain cells, enriching brain networks and opening new routes that your brain can use to bypass damage. Lifelong learning results in a range of positive outcomes, including increased mental and social activity and improved quality of life and wellbeing. It also benefits your brain health. The human brain was built for learning and change so that we can adapt to an ever-changing world. Your brain confers on you the ability to do tomorrow what you couldn't do today. Learning is not just for the young, it is for everyone. Learning is for living and learning is for life. Learning doesn't need to be academic, although it can be.

'Use it or lose it' holds true for the brain. Neglecting mental activities can ultimately lead to brain atrophy and loss of cognitive function. This is because neurons that are left out of action through lack of use become damaged and die and unused branches in your brain are pruned. In contrast, regularly used connections are strengthened. A fit, healthy, dense, well-connected brain is your best defence against brain fog.

Practical tips to exercise your brain

When was the last time you experienced something new or proactively took on a challenge (as opposed to feeling challenged)? If you've been taking the easy road, you can become stuck in a rut and your brain becomes unused to change and unprepared for challenges that may lie ahead. Does this sound familiar? Is it possible that your brain is so understimulated that when real life challenges appear your brain feels overwhelmed?

1. Rediscover the joy of learning

As children, we are driven by curiosity. We ask questions and if the answers don't satisfy our curiosity we ask some more. We interact with the world using all of our senses. We try to figure things out ourselves. When we see something new, we want to try it out. Unfortunately, for many of us, the joy of discovery gets lost to learning by rote and studying for tests and exams. As a consequence, we often associate learning with negative emotions, such as unpleasant stress, failure or even boredom. If we do succeed academically, our satisfaction comes from the reward of exam grades, qualifications, awards or promotions rather than the from the joy of learning.

If you have forgotten the true joy of learning it may be time to reignite your curiosity. Make a list of things that have always fascinated you and promise to learn more about them. Be curious about the world around you. Try looking at things through the eyes of a toddler or a visitor from outer space. Allow yourself the time to wonder how things work or question why we do things the way we do. Ask questions of yourself and of others. Seek answers and knowledge from books, podcasts, or reliable sources via Google. Let yourself be amazed at everyday things. Avoid the cynical shrug, the 'whatever' or the 'who cares'. Test assumptions. Don't limit your world to the familiar. Afford yourself the opportunity to encounter the unfamiliar. Diversify your interests. Don't assume that your viewpoint or worldview is correct; question it, inform it, allow it to evolve. Become curious about other viewpoints, worldviews, cultures, etc. Allow yourself to be amazed by the world and the people around you.

Learning is for life

Make a personal commitment to lifelong learning. Remember neuroplasticity is the brain's ability to change with learning. It can be formal or informal, online or in person, for personal fulfilment or professional advancement. Your chances of success are greater if you choose to learn about something that interests you, something that you enjoy and derive pleasure from. From a personal perspective I can recommend returning to formal education. I understand that returning to full-time education is unlikely to be an option for most people, due to financial or time constraints, but there are many other options to explore and many that are entirely free.

There are hundreds of free Massive Online Open Courses (MOOCs) available from a variety of sources. These courses appeal to multiple tastes and interests; you can study languages, literature, politics, business, culture, science, psychology, nature, history, creative arts, tech, coding and much, much more. Many MOOCs are social learning platforms, which means that the courses enable learning through conversation as well, so people taking the course engage with each other and with the educators through online forums. The online lessons, which usually require a modest time investment (two to three hours per week), take a variety of forms (videos, text, quizzes, etc.). Whether you read up on a topic that interests you, take a night class, join a book club or a historical society, or study for a degree, just make a commitment now to keep on learning. It will bring you joy and your brain will benefit immensely.

2. Create challenge

The key is to set yourself challenges that stretch you but don't push you too far. You want to step just outside your comfort zone. This is something that will be very individual. You are more likely to succeed if you choose something that you enjoy doing or that involves a goal you are motivated to achieve. You can simply choose a new activity that challenges the way you think. Alternatively, if you already engage in a cognitively stimulating activity, why not try to push yourself to the next level? For example, if you play a musical instrument, challenge yourself with a new complex piece that pushes you to the boundaries of your musical ability, commit yourself to a performance or consider learning another instrument. You can apply similar principles to any skills, arts, creative pursuits, sport, hobbies, leisure or intellectual activities.

There is so much hype around brain-training games that I want to take a moment to mention that a recent consensus statement on the brain-training industry from the scientific community states that, while some training produces statistically significant improvement in the specific skill practised during training, claims made promoting brain games are frequently exaggerated and at times misleading. That's not to say that they won't be shown to work at some point in the future, but currently it is important to acknowledge that more research is warranted and findings need to be replicated by independent researchers with no financial interest in the product.

You can, of course, train your brain yourself without commercial games. Any new experience that involves mental effort is likely to bring about changes in the neural systems that support the acquisition of that new skill. Changes will, therefore, occur with computer games but they will also occur with any novel, mentally stimulating activity such as learning a new language, taking up a new musical instrument, creative writing, photography, interior design or finding your way around a new town on holiday. The consensus statement also echoes my own feelings that time spent playing unproven brain-training games is time not spent engaging in other activities such as socialising, exercising and learning, that we know for sure benefit physical, mental and brain health.

Exercise your body

Physical exercise is one of the most important ways to boost brain health and improve brain function. There is no magic pill you can pop to improve your memory but regularly stepping out for a hike or even a brisk walk can nourish your brain. Dancing, gardening and housework will give your brain a boost, too. Physical activity has direct benefits on the structure and functioning of your brain. In contrast, living a sedentary life of physical inactivity can impair your brain function.

Your brain is the most energy demanding organ in your body. Your brain only weighs about 2 per cent of your body but uses 20–25 per cent of your body's energy every day. It costs six calories to run one billion neurons, that's 516 calories out of your daily calorie intake to keep your 86 billion neurons ticking over. Your brain consumes a lot of oxygen and nutrients and needs to be constantly informed of your body's needs and available resources. It depends on its vast neuronal networks to provide that information. Your ability to learn, think and remember is closely linked to your glucose levels and the ability of your brain to efficiently use this energy source.

As I mentioned earlier in this chapter, you need a really healthy cardiovascular system to supply your body and brain with the oxygen and nutrients they need to function. Physical exercise is good for brain function because it helps to maintain the blood flow and the supply of oxygen and nutrients to your brain. Your brain cannot survive for more than a few minutes without oxygen. When you start exercising, the blood flowing to your brain carries extra oxygen and nutrients to your neurons. This increase in oxygen may help to stimulate the production of new brain cells. Physical activity also reduces the risk for cardiovascular disease and stroke which can cause brain fog and severe cognitive impairment.

You're probably familiar with public health recommendations for moderate intensity exercise for thirty minutes five times per week. Remember these recommendations are based on leisure-time physical activity only. You need to do that in addition to the physical activity that you engage in as part of your everyday life and routine. Higher levels of physical activity will bring greater health benefits up to a point. The research that I mentioned earlier, which reported the benefits of doing both aerobic and resistance training, was based on at least moderate activity for forty-five to sixty minutes as many days a week as possible. Physical activity also helps to reduce your brain's exposure to substances that are toxic to the brain. It also lowers the risk of obesity and type-2 diabetes, both of which are conditions associated with brain fog.

It doesn't all have to be about going to the gym and jogging. Think outside the box for ways that you can integrate exercise into your daily routine. Housework counts as moderate exercise, so attack it with gusto. Have fun with it. Play upbeat music in the house while you prepare dinner or do the chores. It's hard to resist the temptation to dance or move in time to the music. Or simply put on your favourite song and dance around your kitchen, bedroom or office.

Physical activity literally changes your brain. It seems to enhance the connections in your brain by stimulating the release of BDNF (brain fertiliser). It also supports your brain cells and helps new ones to grow, which goes some way towards explaining why your brain shrinks less as you age if you remain physically active

Exercising makes your brain more plastic. This means that areas of your brain (such as the hippocampus and prefrontal cortex) are more able to rise to the challenge of learning and, with regular physical exercise, you will see improvements in memory, attention and the speed with which you can process information. Exercise also helps the connections between neurons in your brain to work better. When the emotional centre in your brain (amygdala) and your executive control centre (prefrontal cortex) have strong connections, it becomes easier for you to maintain a healthy weight, for example. This is because this stronger connectivity between these parts of the brain gives you greater control over your impulses and your emotions, including your impulse to eat. Of course, exercise will also keep your weight on track because it burns fat, too. Just think, you can gain these benefits by regularly playing actively with your kids, grandkids, nieces or nephews.

Playing an active sport can make exercise more enjoyable and an element of competition can increase the sense of reward that you experience. Taking up a team sport gives you the added bonus of spending time in the company of others. Find a tennis or golf partner and play together. Getting physically active with friends can increase the enjoyment. You're more likely to stick at it when you have fun.

A growing body of research is starting to show that combining exercise with cognitively demanding activities benefits the brain more than exercise that is not cognitively demanding. While research with mice shows that exercise alone promoted the growth of new neurons in the hippocampus, combining exercise with cognitive demands in a stimulating environment led to more new neurons and neurons that survived for longer. When exercise is combined with something that is cognitively challenging, more BDNF is released than when just exercising. Participating in physical activities that require a combination of cognitive and aerobic tasks could be a way to tap into these added benefits. Learning complex dance or martial arts routines come to mind as examples. I certainly feel cognitively challenged in group aerobic, cross-training or dance classes while learning new steps or routines. Human research shows that collegiate cross-country runners who train extensively on outdoor trails have greater connectivity between brain regions involved in executive function than their sedentary counterparts. Adding a cognitive challenge to your exercise could be as simple as running outdoors instead of on a treadmill in the gym, something that researchers are trying to determine.

Exercise releases 'feel-good' chemicals in the brain called endorphins.

These endorphins improve mood and reduce symptoms of depression, stress and anxiety – all of which contribute to brain fog. Physical activity can also buffer against some of the negative impacts that chronic stress can have on the brain through the reduction of cortisol levels. Maintaining physical fitness will give you more energy to do the things that you want to do, not less. This is particularly important to bear in mind if you feel constantly fatigued. It feels counterintuitive, but exercising will help lift your fatigue. Being active means that you will sleep more soundly too. Exercise tones your brain as well as your butt.

While getting physically active is critical, and will produce noticeable results in your brain performance, it is important to balance exercise with rest and recovery. Sleep, hydration and nutrition are all important aspects of recovery. If you plan to take up resistance training, such as lifting weights, I would recommend that you begin slowly and work under the guidance of an expert to gradually train your body, otherwise you may do yourself more harm than good. You need to restore your body's natural balance by replacing the fluids lost to sweat and you need to eat and sleep to restock on nutrients and energy. Don't become too obsessive about exercising all of the time and don't forget to stretch. Warm up before you exercise; include dynamic stretching before your activity sessions and static stretching afterwards.

While following daily exercise recommendations is good for your body and your brain, it's not the whole story because physical inactivity and a sedentary lifestyle represent health hazards in and of themselves. Exercising for thirty minutes a day is great but what you do for the rest of the day matters too. Do you do a spin class in the morning then sit in front of a computer all day without moving, or perhaps go to the gym after work for an hour then flop in front of a TV for the rest of the evening?

Meeting the recommended physical activity guidelines is not enough. You also need to consider how much time you spend being physically inactive, because too long spent in sedentary behaviour increases your risk for some chronic diseases associated with brain fog. An inactive, sluggish body leads to an inactive, sluggish brain. Physical inactivity is associated with type-2 diabetes and depression. Physical inactivity accelerates the ageing process while physical activity slows it down. The choice is yours to make.

You need to sit less. Prolonged periods of sitting slow down your metabolism, affecting your body's ability to regulate blood pressure, blood sugar and break down body fat, which increases risk of cardiovascular disease, type-2 diabetes and obesity. Even if you are getting your 150 minutes of exercise a week, sitting too much comes with its own risks. On average, in addition to time spent sleeping, we spend seven waking hours every day sitting or lying. How do you compare to the average? We spend the bulk of our days on our butts at a computer, at a desk, watching TV, at the wheel of our car or on a bus, tram or train. Working from home may make matters worse as we do not even have the movement of the commute as part of our daily activity.

Patterns of sedentary behaviour established in childhood persist with age so, in addition to changing your own habits, it's really important to get the kids in your life moving more and sitting less. Adults who report more than four hours a day of screen time are at greater risk of heart attack when compared to adults who log less than two hours a day in front of the TV or other screen-based entertainment. Studies show that obese people sit for two hours and fifteen minutes more per day than lean people. Research suggests that slimmer people in the past actually ate more than we do today but they burned more energy because they were on their feet more. It's not rocket science. You burn on average one calorie per minute sitting, two per minute standing and four per minute walking.

When you park yourself in one spot for hours on end, the lack of movement reduces the flow of blood and the amount of oxygen entering your brain. As a consequence, you may experience a drop in your ability to concentrate. If you slump at your desk with inward drooping shoulders, the hunched position of your body leaves little room for your lungs to expand. Your poor posture shrinks your chest cavity, temporarily limiting the amount of oxygen your lungs can take in. When you sit for long periods of time you don't burn fat as well as you do when you keep moving because prolonged sitting temporarily deactivates the enzyme that breaks down fat. It can also constrict the arteries in your legs, impeding blood flow. This can raise blood pressure and, over time, lead to heart disease which, aside from being an overall health risk, negatively impacts on brain health.

Practical tips to exercise your body

If you are living with one of the many chronic conditions associated with brain fog, you may feel that exercise of any kind is simply beyond you. When every bone in your body is telling you to rest, it is hard to believe that becoming more active will give you more energy, lessen your pain and improve your mood, but it's true. Chronic illness reduces activity levels leading to loss of fitness, fatigue, pain, stiffness, anxiety and depression – exercise counteracts all of these.

Speak to your doctor as they may be able to refer you to occupational or physical therapists who will understand your specific needs and work with you to devise a fitness programme. You will need to start small; the type and amount of exercise you do will depend on the severity of your illness, the amount of pain that you have and whether you have mobility issues or not. Whatever your starting point, you will need to work on your flexibility, strength and endurance (aerobic fitness).

Simple stretching exercises to improve flexibility are a good place to start. In addition to keeping your joints and muscles flexible, stretching reduces pain and stiffness. Yoga and tai chi are excellent for developing flexibility, and stretching is essential as a warm-up for other types of exercise.

If you have been inactive due to chronic illness your muscles will have become deconditioned. With time you will be able to work with weights to build muscle strength, but initially you can begin with moving your arms about, or using them to push to a sitting position in bed; then gradually build your strength so that you can swing your legs to the side to sit on the edge of the bed; then to push yourself to standing from the side of the bed to taking a couple of steps and so on.

Remember, when it comes to building aerobic fitness, every physical activity – including getting dressed, housework and shopping – counts. This will be a very personal journey and you will need to find a balance between building fitness and avoiding post-exertion fatigue or pain; if you would like to go walking, then you may have to give the housework a skip. Your aim is to strengthen your heart and your lungs; this in turn will reduce your fatigue and pain, improve your sleep and build your stamina so that you can gradually become more active – eventually building towards healthy levels of daily exercise.

1. Get physical

We all need to exercise every day. Exercise really is an all-rounder: good for physical, mental and brain health. Exercise can't be optional nor is it a luxury. It is one of the most important things you can do for your brain. Make it a part of your daily routine and you will notice a big difference in your ability to concentrate and other symptoms of brain fog.

You need to build towards doing at least 150 minutes of moderate aerobic activity or seventy-five minutes of vigorous activity each week. Guidelines suggest splitting that over five days, which is good advice, but I wouldn't see that as an excuse to vegetate two days a week. Do some form of physical activity every day. If you don't have a chronic illness but have never exercised before, start with walking – why not try a fifteen-minute walk after dinner this evening?

Don't underestimate the benefits of walking. Regular walkers have been shown to have longer and better-quality sleep than non-walkers. Walking is associated with sharper thinking, enhanced creativity and improved mood. Walking can help boost cognitive function and rejuvenate your brain.

2. Sit less

Break up long spells of sitting with bouts of moving for at least one to two minutes. If your job, like mine, involves extended periods of sitting, get up and walk around at least every two hours if you are a younger adult and every hour if you are an older adult. I'm sure you've often heard people say that they need to take a walk to clear their head. Well it really works. If you come up against a mental block, a walk around the physical block can clear the fog by increasing the flow of glucose and oxygen to your brain.

It's important to avoid long periods of sitting at work or at home in front of a screen. If you work at a desk, don't sit for some of your tasks. For example, you could open your post or take phone calls standing. If colleagues are allowed regular 'smoking breaks' you could consider taking regular walking breaks to reduce your sitting time. Walk rather than sit during your tea or coffee break. After lunch, get up from the table and move about instead of spending your entire lunch break seated.

Avoid long stints sitting in front of the TV, computer or playing console games. If you are struggling to exercise for thirty minutes a day, it's pretty crazy to spend more than an hour or two watching TV every evening. Why not make a pact with yourself to never spend more time watching TV than you spend exercising? Life is precious and short. TV is great, don't get me wrong, I love a good box set myself, but it is a passive activity that doesn't challenge your brain, plus it encourages sedentary behaviour. It's not about cutting it out altogether, it's about balance and making conscious decisions about how you use your precious time. Consider setting limits for yourself in advance. Take conscious note of how much time you are sitting without moving. Get up and move around or go upstairs during the ad breaks, when you finish an episode or when you complete a level of a game. If you follow sport, try standing for some of the game while you watch it on TV; you can pretend you're standing on the side line. If you tend to binge-watch box sets for hours on end, force yourself to get up and walk around for a couple of minutes between each episode. You might find that this will help you to resist the temptation to watch the entire season in one night.

3. Stand tall

Spend more time standing, but don't go overboard. Prolonged standing without opportunities to sit is not good either. The trick is to alternate between the two. Start to view standing as a form of exercise. If you reduced your daily sitting time from eight hours to six hours by standing for two hours, spread over the day, every day for twelve months, the net effect is the equivalent of running six marathons a year. Try to make a point of standing for specific activities like talking on the phone or on your commute to work. However, try not to stand in the same position for long periods and avoid wearing high heels if you do have to stand for prolonged periods.

The brain actually performs better when we stand. In addition to being bad for your health, sitting for prolonged periods can lead to mental fatigue and lack of motion can push your body into sleep mode. Standing desks are a fantastic invention but you don't have to buy one; you can improvise by placing your laptop on a box on your desk. Consider taking meetings or holding conversations while standing.

Watch your posture when you are walking, too: step from heel to toe, using your muscles to hold your tummy and bum in line with the rest of your body. Avoid arching your back and looking down at your feet or at your phone. Make a conscious decision to put your phone in your pocket or your bag before you head out. Take in the world around you. Walking is a great opportunity to feed your senses and paying full attention to your surroundings can be almost meditative. If your physical activity regime includes running, try to keep your head looking forward and try not to bend at the waist, hunch your shoulders or lift your knees too high. Increasing the amount of time that you spend standing and exercising will help you to sleep better.

4. Integrate

Find as many ways as you can to incorporate more movement into your daily routine. Get off the bus or train a couple of stops early. Park a little further away from your destination. Consider walking or cycling to work, if that's a realistic option. Take the stairs as much as possible. Walk while you are on the phone. Walk to talk to a colleague instead of emailing them. Meet friends for a walk rather than for a coffee or brunch. Cut down on screen time and replace it with an active hobby like gardening, DIY, dancing, drumming, hiking, bird-watching or playing sport instead. It really doesn't matter what the hobby is if you enjoy it and it makes you feel good. Consider getting involved in community-based activities, join walking groups, attend dance classes or volunteer for the local beach or park clean-up.

Too often we see exercise as something that we have to do. Another chore, an unpleasant 'grin and bear it' sort of activity. I advise actually grinning while you exercise. This small adjustment can have real benefits. Smiling while you exercise will actually help you to relax, reduce muscle tension, improve the efficiency of your performance and make your workout feel less effortful and more enjoyable.

Key chapter takeaways

- Challenging your brain promotes neuroplasticity.
- Novelty, experiencing new things, new people and new situations, is a critical element of neuroplasticity.

- Learning is like a powerful brain-changing drug that generates new brain cells, enriches brain networks and opens new routes which the brain can use to bypass damage.
- Use it or lose it. Neurons that are left out of action through lack of use become damaged and die.
- Exercise helps to maintain the blood flow and the supply of oxygen and nutrients to the brain.
- Physical activity also helps to reduce the brain's exposure to neurotoxins.
- Physical exercise gives rise to the growth of new neurons in the hippocampus and also helps the connections between neurons to work better.
- Physical inactivity is associated with depression, diabetes and a number of other chronic conditions that, in turn, are associated with brain fog.
- Physical inactivity accelerates the ageing process while physical activity slows it down.

Get ready for the 30-day plan

- If you engage in regular exercise, go to https://bit.ly/HSE_Exercise for a refresher on how to exercise safely, different levels of intensity and suggestions for various types of exercise.
- If you haven't exercised in a while, go to https://www.nhs.uk/live-well/exercise/ to download a booklet that will help you to determine an exercise plan most appropriate to your current fitness level.
- Root out your sports gear and make sure it's clean and comfortable. You don't want to scupper your chances of success before you even start because you can't find your kit.
- If your sports gear is past its sell-by date, consider investing in some new gear. It doesn't have to be expensive or fancy. The main thing is that it's comfortable and fit for purpose, especially footwear.
- Dust off any sports equipment that you will need and check it's safe and working properly.

Change: Nutrition

What is brain fuel?

When you shop for food, cook or order from a menu, do you consider the impact on your brain? Chances are you don't. Most likely you'll consider your likes, dislikes, cravings, hunger level, mood and world view or life philosophy. Depending on your weight, health and motivation, you might also consider the calories, fat, sugar, gluten, allergies, additives and preservatives. Next time you shop for food, I suggest you consider shopping for your brain.

Your brain requires a constant supply of fuel. That fuel comes from the food you eat; what you eat directly affects your brain and how well it functions. If you choose your food carefully it will pay dividends upstairs, so you can eat your way to a better brain. The phrase 'you are what you eat' counts for your brain too!

Your brain is a thirsty organ. It needs to be kept hydrated to function properly. Your brain is made up of 73 per cent water with the remainder made up of macronutrients (fat, protein and carbohydrates) and micronutrients (vitamins and minerals) that impact on your brain development, your brain functioning, your energy and your mood.

Nutrients

Adopting a healthy diet is the best way to get the nutrients that your body and brain need. When it comes to brain health, multivitamins are no substitute for a healthy diet. There is insufficient evidence that multivitamins or other supplements improve brain health in adults without a diagnosed deficiency. Vitamin B12 and folate deficiency can impair cognitive function and people who are deficient will benefit from supplementation. However, there is no convincing evidence to recommend daily supplementation in healthy adults whose levels are within the recommended range. If you think you may be deficient, visit your doctor for testing. Do not take any 'brain health' supplement without first consulting your doctor. While many vitamins and minerals are essential in small doses for brain health and health in general, they can be harmful if taken to excess. The quality of the ingredients in supplements vary widely and could even contain harmful ingredients. I urge you to take the often vague and exaggerated claims made on supplement packaging with a pinch of salt. It's big business; the global dietary supplement market was valued at 140 billion dollars in 2018. Please don't spend a penny on supplements to boost your brain health – invest your money in good quality fresh food instead. You can get all the nutrients that you need from a Mediterranean diet. Here's all you need to know about brain-healthy nutrients.

Fats

While you need some fat in your diet the type of fat you consume is of critical importance to your overall health. Limiting your fat intake to monounsaturated and polyunsaturated fats is the healthiest option. Steer clear of trans fats as there are no known health benefits; in fact they have been banned in a number of countries. Eating trans fats increases harmful cholesterol and reduces beneficial cholesterol. For every 2 per cent of calories that you get from trans fats you increase your risk of heart disease by 23 per cent. Trans fats, found in baked goods, fried food, margarine and frozen pizza for example, increase inflammation and contribute to insulin resistance. Researchers at Harvard found that women who ate the most saturated fats, from meat and butter for example, had the worst cognitive performance;

while women who ate the most monounsaturated, fats from olive oil and nuts for example, did the best. Researchers suspect that the inflammation caused by the saturated fat consumption leads to damage in the arteries in the brain which, in turn, impairs cognitive functioning.

The brain cannot burn fat for energy, so it has no use for saturated fats. Instead, your brain needs omega-3 and omega-6, which are polyunsaturated fats. If you become deficient in omega-3 you will likely experience memory problems, fatigue, mood swings and depression. Omega-3 fatty acids are essential for brain function and critical for maintaining the health of your brain cells. These fatty acids can also reduce inflammation, which is linked to brain fog. Your body can't make omega-3 fatty acids so you must get them from the food you eat. Foods rich in omega-3 include cold-water fatty fish (e.g. salmon, mackerel, tuna, sardines), nuts and seeds (e.g. walnuts, chia seeds, flax seeds) and some plant oils (e.g. canola oil, flaxseed oil). Some foods (e.g. certain brands of yogurt, juices, milk, infant formula) have been fortified with omega-3 – check the labels. The NHS recommend increasing omega-3 intake by eating at least two portions of fish a week.

Omega-6 is also important; however, most Western diets include way too much omega-6. Some American diets include a ratio of omega-6 to omega-3 as high as 30:1. A healthy ratio of omega-6 to omega-3 should be closer to 2:1. To bring your omega-6 consumption down you need to ditch the processed food and takeaways and avoid peanuts, corn, fatty foods such as bacon and chicken skin and vegetable oil from canola.

Artificial trans fats are the devil, avoid them like the plague. You'll need to play detective at first to weed them out of your diet because they sneak in everywhere, especially in processed, packaged foods. My preference is to give processed foods a wide berth altogether but if that's not an option for you, you'll need to read the labels and ditch anything containing trans fats which might be labelled as hydrogenated fats, partially hydrogenated fats, shortening, DATEM, monoglycerides or diglycerides. If reading ingredients isn't your thing, then avoid dough-nuts, cakes, pies, biscuits, crackers, frozen pizza base, margarine and creamy spreads. Sorry!

Cholesterol

Cholesterol is a steroid that is essential for human health and brain function. It forms the building blocks for hormones, including cortisol, testosterone and oestrogens. Your liver and your brain both manufacture cholesterol. Your liver can produce all of the cholesterol that your body needs to carry out its many essential functions and can generally maintain a healthy level of blood cholesterol. The brain uses cholesterol to manufacture the myelin sheaths that surround the communication cables, which ensure the speedy transmission of neural signals. The brain has the highest cholesterol content of any organ in your body. It manufactures its own supply because the cholesterol made in the liver cannot traverse the blood brain barrier. You *don't* need to add foods containing cholesterol to your diet.

Protein

To function properly, your brain and nervous system also need an adequate supply of amino acids found in protein-rich foods. These amino acids are the raw materials used to make neurotransmitters, the chemical messengers that carry signals throughout your brain. Amino acids, the building blocks of the protein that you eat, are essentially the precursors of neurotransmitters. For example, protein-rich foods like turkey, soy, eggs, dairy and legumes contain an amino acid called tyrosine. When you eat any of these proteins, enzymes in your body can turn the amino acid tyrosine into the neurotransmitter dopamine, which is involved in a variety of brain functions including memory, attention, mood, reward and sleep.

Vitamins and minerals

Your brain also benefits from trace minerals, B vitamins and antioxidants.[26] Minerals like iron, copper, zinc and sodium in the right proportions are essential for brain health and cognitive development.

Iron has many vital functions in your body, including transporting and storing oxygen and energy metabolism. Your brain gets a great boost from iron because it needs oxygen to work well. Blood carries vital oxygen supplies to your brain cells and that process needs iron.

Iron-deficient anaemia is a condition where your body doesn't have enough red blood cells. Brain fog, mental fatigue and tiredness can occur if red blood cells cannot deliver sufficient oxygen to the body's tissues and organs, including the brain. There are several forms of anaemia, each with a different cause. Iron-deficient anaemia is the most common form; other types can be caused by lack of vitamin B12 or folate in your body. Anaemia can be related to an illness such as systemic lupus erythematosus (SLE). Anaemia is also a common side-effect of cancer treatments and can be caused by some cancers.

Vitamin B12 plays a critical role in making and maintaining the myelin sheaths that protect your brain's communication cables, ensuring fast and effective transmission of neural signals. Your body can't make vitamin B12 so you must get it from meat, eggs, poultry, dairy or other animal products. If you are vegetarian or vegan you are at risk of Vitamin B12 deficiency unless you eat foods which have been fortified with B12. If you become deficient in B12, you may experience symptoms of brain fog such as memory issues and difficulty thinking and reasoning. Coeliac disease and Crohn's disease interfere with nutritional absorption and if you have either condition you could be deficient. As we age, changes to our digestive tract may decrease the amount of vitamin B12 that is absorbed. In addition, levels of B12 might also be reduced simply because we tend to eat less in later life.

If you suspect you may be deficient in iron or B12 speak to your doctor about having your levels tested. Iron deficiency can be treated by upping your dietary intake of iron or through supplements. Foods rich in iron include: meat, green leafy vegetables, beans, nuts, apricots, prunes, raisins and foods fortified with iron. Bear in mind that some foods (e.g. tea, coffee, milk, wholegrain cereals) and some medications (antacids and proton pump inhibitors) can make it more difficult for your body to absorb iron. Daily supplementation or vitamin B12 injections are a safe and easy way to address a B12 deficiency and reverse the associated cognitive symptoms.

Don't buy into the market that's trying to get you to purchase supplements to boost your memory. It is far better to get the nutrients that your brain needs from healthy fresh food; you don't need supplements unless your doctor says you are deficient.

Antioxidants

Antioxidants, mainly found in fruit and vegetables, play an important role in preventing cell damage by neutralising free radicals that have the capacity to damage and destroy brain cells. Antioxidants are like damage-limitation specialists. The principle antioxidant micronutrients are beta-carotene, vitamin C and vitamin E. The body can't manufacture these micronutrients so they must be obtained through diet. Plant-based foods such as fruits, vegetables, whole grains, nuts, seeds, herbs and spices are the best sources of antioxidants.

Glucose

Your brain is a high-energy consumer. Your digestive system converts the carbohydrates (sugars and starches) in the food you eat into glucose, which is absorbed by your stomach and small intestine and then released into your bloodstream. Your brain relies almost exclusively on glucose as its energy source. When your brain needs energy, glucose can easily pass through the blood brain barrier to satisfy the energy demands of billions of your brain cells, which use about one fifth of the oxygen and glucose circulating in your blood at any one time. While most of this fuel is used for neural communication, about a third is needed for the essential housekeeping that keeps your brain cells healthy and your brain tissue alive.

Without enough glucose in the brain, communication between neurons can break down because neurotransmitters are not produced. When neural communication breaks down, brain fog symptoms are likely to emerge. When your blood sugar is low you'll probably experience brain fog and have a cracking headache. The trick is to make sure that your brain always has an adequate supply of glucose while keeping your blood sugar stable. The best way to do that is to eat complex carbohydrates such as whole wheat and brown rice rather than simple carbohydrates like honey or fruit juice concentrate that provide quick energy and a glucose spike. Complex carbohydrates provide time-released energy with less spike because they are hard for your body to break down. Doughnuts, cakes, white foods and pasta are not smart foods to eat if you want to banish brain fog. Sorry, again!

The glycaemic load of any food refers to how quickly it raises blood sugar in relation to the amount of fibre it contains. Fibre is important because it lowers the effect that the food has on insulin. Good sources of high-fibre, complex carbohydrates include: sweet potatoes, turnips, berries, grapefruit, carrots, butternut squash, legumes (e.g. lentils, beans) and whole grains.

. Low glucose levels (hypoglycaemia), a complication of diabetes, are associated with poor cognitive function and problems with attention. The frontal lobes are so sensitive to reductions in glucose that altered mental function is a primary signal of glucose deficiency. Diets that are high in sugars can cause oxidative stress and have been associated with impaired brain function. Eating a balanced diet rich in vitamins, minerals and antioxidants can protect your brain from oxidative stress.

Water

Your brain is comprised mainly of water. You need it in your blood to transport oxygen. Generally speaking, we don't drink enough fluids. When your brain has a full reserve of water you will be able to focus and think faster and more clearly. Water is also essential for the transportation of nutrients. In the absence of proper hydration, nutrients and oxygen may not be delivered efficiently, with knock-on effects on brain function. Make sure that you consume enough fluids every day so that your brain is kept hydrated and properly serviced with the energy and nutrients that it needs to function well. Remember you need water to remove toxins, including toxic waste, from your brain too. We're often told to drink eight glasses of water per day but that is overly simplistic. A better rule of thumb is to divide your weight in pounds by two and aim for that many fluid ounces of water each day.

Drink fluids before, during and after exercise. Make sure you drink more in hot weather to take account of fluid lost to sweating. An increase in the frequency of urination or any other change in your usual pattern may signify an infection. Don't be tempted to reduce your fluid intake to reduce urinary frequency or urgency as this may lead to dehydration, especially if you have a kidney or urinary tract infection. Keep hydrated and if frequent urination is an issue, make an appointment to visit your doctor and follow their advice.

Practical tips to nourish your brain

1. Go Mediterranean

Instead of going to the shop with a list of all the macro- and micro-nutrients that your brain requires, take a big-picture approach and keep your brain in good shape by adopting a Mediterranean-style diet.

The Mediterranean diet is a healthy and sustainable eating plan that promotes heart health and prevents chronic disease. One important aspect of the Mediterranean diet is that meals are social events shared with family and friends. Diet and lifestyle choices that are good for your heart are also good for your brain because your brain depends on a healthy cardiovascular system to function well.

To follow a Mediterranean diet you need to consume vegetables, fruits, whole grains, nuts, seeds and olive oil daily. Eat fish, poultry, beans and eggs weekly and limit your consumption of red meat. You can eat dairy products in moderation. Healthy unsaturated fats, eaten instead of saturated and trans fats, are a mainstay of a Mediterranean diet. There are two types of unsaturated fats – monounsaturated and polyunsaturated. Olive oil, a monounsaturated fat, is the primary source of fat eaten on a Mediterranean diet.

The Mediterranean diet also emphasises foods that are rich in omega-3 fatty acids, including whole grains, fresh fruits and vegetables, fish and garlic. Omega-3 fatty acids help reduce inflammation. In contrast, when consumed to excess, most omega-6 fatty acids tend to promote inflammation. The Mediterranean diet has a healthier balance between omega-3 and omega-6 fatty acids than other Western diets. A varied diet that is rich in antioxidants (e.g. fruits, vegetables and nuts) comes with the added bonus that these foods tend to be high in fibre, low in choles-terol, low in saturated fat and a good source of vitamins and minerals.

Vegetarians adopting a Mediterranean diet can avoid a deficit in protein by eating a varied diet that includes nuts, seeds, beans, eggs and high-protein whole grains such as quinoa.

In terms of food, what you put into your mouth affects what comes out of your brain. So make sure you know what you're eating. Where possible try to cook from scratch, use fresh ingredients and avoid processed foods. If you must eat processed or pre-packaged food read the labels and choose carefully, watch out for saturated fats.

Your brain enjoys nothing more than breathing in plenty of oxygen as you exercise, but to redeem the benefits of all that movement you need a good supply of iron running through your veins. This means topping up on foods such as green leafy vegetables like spinach, fortified cereal, pulses and meat.

Choose your fluids wisely. You might also want to avoid drinking tea with meals as it prevents the uptake of iron. Avoid fluids that contain added sugar or caffeine. Go easy on the alcohol too. Heavy drinking is harmful to brain health. Drinking alcohol will also affect your weight and impair your sleep.

2. Maintain a healthy weight

If you want to optimise your brain function you need to maintain a healthy weight. Depending on your age, being overweight or being underweight can have a negative impact on how well your brain works. Obesity is associated with brain atrophy, which means that it is linked with the loss of brain cells and brain connections.

Body mass index (BMI) is a measure that uses your height and your weight to work out if your weight is healthy. High BMI, or unhealthy weight, is linked with reduced brain volume. If you lose brain volume you will lose brain function. High BMI is specifically associated with loss of brain cells and the connections between them in areas of the brain involved in memory and critical thinking. Obesity and high BMI are linked to several health issues including high blood pressure and type-2 diabetes which are associated with cognitive dysfunction. This makes it difficult to disentangle the link between obesity and impaired brain function from the link between impaired cognitive function and conditions that are related to obesity. Nonetheless, obesity is a risk factor for impaired functions associated with the frontal lobes (e.g. executive function and working memory) and the hippocampus (learning and memory).

Those who are obese can experience a reduction in a particular protein that protects against inflammation, leading to a chronic inflammatory state and metabolic disease, both of which effect brain function and are associated with brain fog. The brains of people who are obese in middle age are ten years 'older' than the brains of those who are not obese. Research suggests that middle age may represent a critical period for brain ageing, where vulnerability to obesity is particularly acute compared with later life.

The key is to identify your ideal weight, attain it and maintain it. If you are trying to maintain a healthy weight, it is important to remember that small changes can make big differences. Even something simple like changing the colour or size of your plate can reduce the amount of food you consume at one sitting. Have a snack-free day or a sugar-free one. Or try reducing your portion sizes by 10 per cent. Serve a smaller portion, eat, then wait a few minutes. If you are still hungry get some more but you may well find that you are actually no longer hungry. Make sure that you eat regularly. When you eat regularly you are more likely to feel satisfied and eat appropriate portions than if you allow yourself to get too hungry.

Aim to spend longer preparing your food than you do eating it. If your diet is too high in calories it can increase your risk of memory loss. In fact, people who eat more than 2,000 calories a day have double the risk of memory loss compared to people who eat fewer than 1,500 calories. Simply replacing some high-calorie sugary snacks with a healthy alternative could help you hold on to memory function in later life.

Try to be more aware of when you are eating to see whether you might be able to identify why you are actually eating. It may be that you are eating out of stress, or boredom or anxiety. Becoming aware of the times you eat when you're not physically hungry can give you the impetus to change unhealthy eating habits – more on this in Chapter 11. If you are eating because of anxiety then try to address the cause of the anxiety or any other emotional reasons.

When you are sleep deprived, you are less able to resist temptation and you are likely to experience increased hunger and appetite due to elevated levels of endocannabinoids. You are also likely to eat unhealthy snacks and consume more between meals. If you are serious about losing weight you will also need to make sure that you are getting enough sleep.

Getting physically active will help with weight loss, plus it's good for your brain and your heart. Exercising doesn't just burn calories, it also strengthens connections in your brain in a way that gives you greater control over your impulses and emotions, including your impulse to eat. Get active to resist the temptation to eat junk.

3. Balance your microbiota

There are a number of simple things that you can do to build a healthier microbiota. You might be surprised to learn that exercise is one of those things. Walking for one kilometre (e.g. fifteen minutes) will help to balance your microbes. Making sure you have enough fibre in your diet is another. Most of us don't eat enough fibre – women should aim for about 25 grams of fibre a day and men 38 grams, as this feeds the 'good guy' gut bacteria. Fibre is also a great way to keep constipation at bay and some types can lower blood sugar levels too.

Stock up on fibre-filled fruit and vegetables and get in the habit of eating them daily. Pretty much all veggies are high in fibre – artichokes are the star of the show but you'll get fibre from broccoli, brussels sprouts, carrots, kale and spinach. Avocados are packed with fibre as are raspberries. Other fruits that contain fibre include apples and pears. Before you know it, you'll be craving these healthy sources of fibre.

If you do find yourself craving unhealthy snacks like cakes, chocolate and doughnuts, choose raspberries, strawberries or blueberries instead. Stick with these substitutions for a while and you will find that it gets easier as your microbiota gets healthier. Make sure you mix things up when it comes to food. We are all creatures of habit and despite access to almost any type of food imaginable we tend to self-limit and stick with our favourites, our comfort foods. Most of us just alternate the same few dinners and lunches. But by introducing variety into your diet you can prevent a dominant microbe from bullying you into unhealthy food choices.

Key chapter takeaways

- What you eat directly affects your brain and how well it functions.
- Omega-3 fatty acids are important for brain performance and memory and can reduce inflammation.

- Your body produces all of the cholesterol that it needs. You *don't* need to add foods containing cholesterol to your diet.
- Iron and B12 are essential for healthy brain function. If you think you may be deficient speak to your doctor about getting tested.
- Keep your brain hydrated. When your brain has a full reserve of water you will be able to focus and think faster and more clearly.
- Obesity and high-BMI are associated with cognitive dysfunction.
- To keep your brain in good shape, adopt a Mediterranean diet and maintain a healthy weight.
- Balance your microbiota through exercise and a high fibre diet.

Get ready for the 30-day plan

- Remove any unhealthy foods from your cupboards, fridge and freezer. Go through them one by one. Read ingredients and remove all items that:
  - are overly processed,*
  - contain added sugar or added salt,
  - are out of date.
- Limit the impact of endocrine disrupting compounds; see advice in Chapter 3.

You don't have to do this all at once, just do your best. Every little helps. One step at a time will work perfectly well once you continue to take steps.

---

* Food processing takes many forms, including freezing, canning, baking and drying. Not all processed foods are bad for you. Some foods, like milk for example, have to be processed to make them safe. Many processed foods are highly calorific and have additives including fat, salt and sugar to make them taste better or last longer on the shelf. When comparing foods with helpful traffic light colour coding labels, you need to choose greens and ambers and avoid reds. If you have to read the label, then you need to choose foods that are low in sugar (5g or less per 100g), salt (.3g of salt or .1g of sodium), total fat (3g or less per 100g) and saturated fats (1.5g or less per 100g).

Part Four
Future

Have a unique plan.

The Art of War – Sun Tzu

Future:
30-Day Plan

Knowledge is power. By changing your behaviour you can make your future brain fog-free. This 30-day plan is designed to help you to cultivate brain-healthy habits to clear your brain fog and transform your life. There is nothing you can't do once you get your habits right. It will be tough at first but if you stick with the plan, which is really a 30-day habit modification programme, living a brain-healthy life will become effortless and automatic – because that's the nature of habits.

A word about habits

Throughout our lives we all make choices that eventually become habits. Some of these habits are beneficial to our health and some are not. There is no getting away from the fact that some of our habitual choices – particularly around sleep, stress, exercise and diet – may contribute to our brain fog. Through reading this book, you have acquired knowledge of your symptoms, your brain, your biology and the behaviours that could be contributing to your brain fog. Your mission over the next thirty days is to make new choices and develop new routines to eradicate or at the very least minimise your brain fog symptoms. Understanding how your unhelpful habits were formed will help you to overcome, replace or change them. I'm not pretending that this will be easy but it is possible and the payoff – reclaiming your brain and your 'self' – is well worth the effort.

Habits are the result of your brain's need to be efficient and economical with its limited energy supplies. Let's go back to Tim, his bran flakes and his blood test from earlier in the book. Several years ago, Tim saw an ad on the TV saying that bran flakes were fortified with vitamins and good for keeping your bowels regular. Tim liked the sound of that. He'd been feeling a bit run down and his bowels were slimy and sluggish. Next time Tim went to the supermarket he bought a box of bran flakes. He opted for the large box because it was much better value than the small box. He thought they tasted a bit like cardboard but they weren't awful. He said, 'I figured if they helped to move my sluggish bowel along then I can live with the bland taste. Anyway, they don't taste too bad with a couple of spoons of sugar on top.' Tim didn't actually notice any difference to his bowel movements but he hates to waste food and so decided to continue having them for breakfast till the large box was gone. Soon he was automatically reaching for the bran flakes with milk and sugar each morning. Long before the box was finished, this new pattern of behaviour was automated by Tim's brain and bran flakes with milk and sugar became his breakfast habit.

Your brain doesn't distinguish between good or bad habits or whether habits achieve the purpose of your original choice or not. Your brain just looks for patterns that can be automated in order to make the most efficient use of neural resources. Once a habit is formed, your thinking brain is no longer involved in making a choice or decision about that behaviour because it has relinquished control to your pattern-loving basal ganglia. Once a habit is established, changing or replacing it is effortful. Habits stick and can re-emerge even if they haven't been used regularly in a while. Generally speaking, this makes sense because, for example, you don't want to have to relearn how to tie shoe laces when you've spent the summer in sandals. To replace an old, unhelpful habit you will initially have to work hard to fight the brain's tendency to automate; but once you put in the work repeating the new behaviour each day, the new helpful behaviour itself becomes a habit and will, by definition, be effortless. Behaviours become habits through repetition.

Let's say we decide to change things up a bit for the rats in the habit lab in MIT. We swap the loud click for a bell, we keep the screen and the T-maze but this time we place the chocolate in the right corner of the T rather than the left corner. As with the initial experiment, over time, with repetition, the rats will learn to sprint up the aisle and hang a sharp right as soon as the bell tolls and the screen lifts. Then one day we decide to replace the bell with the original loud click. What happens? The rats run up the aisle and hang an immediate left. The old habit is still there. It is critical that you remember this as you work through the 30-day plan. Your old patterns will still be there lurking in the background but you can take control and make new choices that will, with conscious effort and regular repetition, become new habits that force the old ones into the deep recesses of your brain.

Deconstructing how habits work will help you to disrupt and reconstruct the new habits that will help to alleviate your brain fog symptoms. First, there is the trigger (e.g. loud click or bell) that tells the brain to go into automatic mode and which habit to use (e.g. turn left or turn right). Then there is the routine (e.g. run down aisle and turn left or run down aisle and turn right) and finally there is the reward (chocolate) which tells your brain whether this particular sequence of events is worth remembering or repeating.

Over time, with repetition, this sequence 'trigger, routine, reward' becomes more and more automatic. The trigger and the reward become entwined and a sense of anticipation emerges, cravings develop and a habit is generated. Once embedded in your brain, habits never really disappear and can be reactivated at any time. Indeed, they are more likely to be reactivated at times of stress. This is one of the reasons this 30-day plan prioritises stress management. Sleep is also prioritised not only because of its relationship with stress but also because poor sleep makes it more likely that we will fall into old unhealthy habits.

For the rats, the trigger was a sound. Your triggers, also known as cues, will take many forms. They can be something visual like seeing a chocolate bar as you go to pay for your groceries, the smell of vinegar on chips, an ad on the radio, the sound of ice clinking in a glass, a time of day, a place, a person, a group of people, an event, a mood, an emotion or even a thought. Routines can be really simple or quite convoluted, from reaching for the bran flakes, opening the fridge, pouring milk and sprinkling sugar to a much more complex series of actions, like those involved when you stick your key in the ignition and drive to work completely on autopilot.

Chocolate was the reward for the rats and is indeed a reward for many of us humans. Rewards can take several forms – food, alcohol, praise, purchases, physical sensations, emotional feelings or a sense of achievement. The aim of this 30-day plan is to deliberately design new brain-healthy habits but it is important to know that habits can also emerge without our permission. Being conscious, aware and actively monitoring your triggers, routines, rewards and everyday behaviours is critical to success. You will probably find this exhausting – after all, this kind of conscious awareness and active decision-making is resource heavy. In fact, it is exactly what your brain is trying to avoid through resource-light habitual behaviours. But with time and repetition your brain will see the pattern as an opportunity to make more efficient use of resources by transforming the exhausting behaviour into an automated habitual one.

The extra effort is only required in the short term; once your new healthy habits emerge they will become as effortless as your old ones. The good news is that even small shifts can change a pattern. Awareness is the greatest weapon against unwanted habits. By becoming attuned to your triggers and rewards you will gain insight into how you can change your routines. Becoming aware of your habitual behaviours can be very enlightening. We do so much on autopilot without question that just asking yourself why you do X, Y, or Z can be very revealing and can help you to determine whether a particular habit is actually a choice that you would make today or a hangover from your past. You will find that many of these habits were established a long time ago, when you were a child even. You may not even recall why you behave in that way or why you made the original choice.

In order to make habits stick, you need to choose a simple trigger and a clearly defined reward. People who successfully embed healthy habits, such as regular exercise, tend to choose a specific trigger, such as exercising first thing in the morning, and identify a reward. It really is very personal. Sharon loves how completing a workout at lunchtime clears her head and makes her feel sharp for the afternoon. Dave looks forward to his big bowl of hot porridge after walking the dogs in the park. Just days into her new running routine, Bonnie begins to crave the endorphins that are released when she goes for her run at 7 a.m.

As you work through this programme, you will need to pick triggers and rewards that work for you. Each new routine that you aim to turn into a healthy habit will need to be sandwiched between a trigger and a reward. Your chances of success increase when your new routine is bookended between familiar things. The secret to changing a habit is to use the same triggers and rewards but change the routine.

Cravings power the trigger–reward neural sequence. Once craving enters the equation, it becomes more difficult to break the habit sequence because we associate the trigger with the reward to the extent that we begin to anticipate it. If your mum always serves you a steaming hot bowl of homemade soup when you visit her on Wednesday evenings, you will start to anticipate the soup on the bus journey there and will be quite disappointed if there is no soup when you arrive. You might even let the lack of soup colour the tone of your visit with your mum. If the reward that we anticipate is not forthcoming, our desire is denied and we feel frustrated, angry, deprived and disappointed. This is one of the reasons that habits are so powerful. Desire can become an obsessive, addiction-like craving that drives automatic behaviour even when we know the harm that it can do to our health, lives and relationships.

Cravings are powerful but thankfully there are mechanisms that you can employ to overcome them. A first step is to identify the craving. Becoming aware of it will help you to take action to ignore the temptation. For longer-term goals like losing weight, successful dieters will envisage a specific long-term goal like fitting into an outfit for a friend's wedding.

When my first book came out, I found myself doing a lot of travel, sometimes to multiple countries in the same week. I found it hard to fit in exercise and also found it very easy to eat way more than I normally would. When December came round I realised that I had gained 6kg. In January, I was invited to appear on *Home and Family* on the Hallmark Channel in California. For someone like me with no profile in the US, this was huge. I was so excited but I was keen to get back to my ideal weight. I set myself a goal to lose the weight before my appearance on the show on 24 February. Time was tight. But my desire to be in good shape for that TV appearance was so strong that it allowed me to resist all snacks, eat only healthy food, walk endless miles and go to the gym four times a week. By the time 24 February came round I'd lost 5kg and was starting to look toned. Without that specific goal I know I wouldn't have attained the weight loss in the same timeframe.

It is also important to have a signal that the activity in which you are engaging, the soon-to-become healthy habit, is working. I stood on the scales every day and was rewarded by gradual weight loss. I know the recommendation is to weigh yourself once a week but I'm impatient and the daily weigh-in motivated me. I also found it motivating to track my exercise on my iWatch. Essentially, I cultivated a craving – to lose weight – and pursued it obsessively.

It is relatively simple to cultivate a craving. For example, you want to work on going to bed at a regular time every night. Let's say you pick 11 p.m. as your trigger. You might decide to reinforce that by setting an alarm on your phone. You have decided that your reward for going to bed at 11 p.m. each night is to apply your favourite body lotion before getting into bed. You can cultivate a craving for the smell and sensation of that body lotion by thinking about it throughout the day and by reminding yourself of the reward that awaits you at bedtime. By anticipating the reward, you can cultivate a craving to drive the habit loop of getting up off the sofa to go to bed at 11 p.m.

One of the key activities on the first day of the 30-day plan is choosing the cravings that you will build on or cultivate. You will be working on developing multiple habits around sleep and exercise and diet and each will have their own trigger–routine–reward sequence.

You may want to be more precise than attempting to cultivate a craving such as 'being brain fog free'. Research has shown that we respond better to specific targets with clear outcomes. Of course, being free of brain fog is the ultimate goal, but you are more likely to reach that goal if you break it down into steps. I recommend that you focus on the things you miss most from your pre-brain fog life. Olive wants to be able to tell funny jokes again; Amanda wants to be able to make spaghetti bolognaise without having to consult a recipe; Patsy wants to be able to follow the plot so she can watch TV with her son again. This will be very personal to you.

In order to change an existing habit you need to understand and address the craving. To recap, you keep the same triggers and rewards, change the routine and cultivate a craving. When I first learned about this, I thought, hold on a second, how does that work if the reward is unhealthy? Charles Duhigg gives the best explanation I've come across in his excellent book *The Power of Habit*. Duhigg says that Alcoholics Anonymous succeeds because it uses the same triggers and the same rewards to feed the craving but changes the routine. Alcoholics, Duhigg explains, crave a drink, not necessarily because it makes them drunk or because they crave oblivion but rather because they want to forget, escape, relax, blunt feelings or because they crave company. AA forces alcoholics to change their routine by getting them to come to meetings when they crave a drink. At these meetings they can relax in company and talk through their feelings which gives them relief and the payoff they were actually craving.

So the take-home message is that habits and cravings are complicated and we shouldn't assume the most obvious. For example, don't take it for granted that you snack because you are hungry or binge on Netflix because the show is too brilliant not to. Probe your behaviour more deeply. Do you snack at work because you are hungry or because you are bored? Do you binge on Netflix because you want to relax or because you want to dampen down feelings of loneliness or anxiety? Keep probing until you find what you really crave.

Rewarding yourself is absolutely critical to success. Give yourself gold stars, congratulate yourself on every achievement and keep track of your progress. Even checking a mark on a list is rewarding. I couldn't live without my to-do list. First of all, it gets all the potential stressors, the things that I need to do, out of my head and onto a page where I can prioritise them and give them a deadline date. Second of all, I get huge, and I mean huge, satisfaction out of checking an item off my list. I get terribly disappointed if I go to check an item off my list only to discover I hadn't added it in the first place! Truth be told, I've often added it so that I can mark it as complete in my Excel file. It might seem ridiculous but it is both rewarding and motivating and works for me.

Make sure that you get the level of 'to do' right, though. I'd never put 'write a book' on my to-do list. That's a goal, not an action. I would, however, break down the tasks that take me a step closer to that goal, for example, 'research content for Chapter 4', 'decide on key messages for Chapter 5', 'write practical tips for Chapter 6' and so on. Essentially, I am engineering opportunities for early success, which lifts my mood, eliminates the 'I have to write a book' stress which can be overwhelming and gives me a greater sense of control and satisfaction.

Your brain was built to adapt and change. Having read this book, you are armed with the knowledge that you need to understand your brain fog and yourself. Adopting brain-healthy habits is the most powerful way to beat brain fog. This 30-day programme will help you to beat brain fog and build a brighter, brain-healthy future. Things will get better – not all at once but a bit at a time.

Studies show that people who believe that change is possible are more likely to attain the changes that they strive for. What you do, what you think and what you believe are all important ingredients for success. Social support and success go hand in hand, so recruit supportive friends and/or family. Consider seeking support from different people for different habits that you are working on. Would your best friend or a work colleague walk with you every day or join you in the gym? Would your partner help keep you on the straight and narrow when it comes to implementing your new sleep routine? Working with groups like Weight Watchers or joining in a Parkrun can be really motivating.

Rewards don't have to be external things like food, shopping or holidays; they can be internal feelings, sensations and emotions. Understanding your motivations will help you to plan in a way that increases your likelihood of successful habit change. Psychologists divide motivation into extrinsic and intrinsic. Engaging in a behaviour or activity to gain a reward or indeed to avoid punishment is extrinsically motivated. In contrast, intrinsic motivation refers to engaging in a behaviour because you find it personally rewarding. If you play a sport to win trophies, you are extrinsically motivated. If you do it because you have fun and find it really enjoyable you are intrinsically motivated. Tidying the house before your mother visits to avoid her criticism is also extrinsic motivation where you do it to avoid something unpleasant. In contrast, tidying your house because you enjoy it is intrinsic. Studying to get a good grade is extrinsic (external to you). Studying because you find the material fascinating is intrinsic (internal to you). It doesn't take an expert to understand that intrinsic motivation is the ideal – it is far easier to do something that you find enjoyable. But that's not always possible; you may simply have zero desire to engage in exercise or you might even find it unpleasant. This is where extrinsic motivation comes in useful.

As you complete the 30-day plan, your behaviour will be driven by both internal and external motivators. Providing exclusively external rewards for all of the healthy behaviours you are trying to turn into habits won't work and actually might be counterproductive. Reserve extrinsic rewards for behaviours in which you have no intrinsic interest. If you absolutely hate exercise then reward yourself. Make a delicious smoothie after your jog or watch an episode of your favourite series after the gym. The extrinsic reward will incentivise you to engage in the healthful behaviour. The good news is that as you learn the new behaviour, you may become intrinsically motivated to engage in it – in other words, you might actually start to enjoy going to the gym. Receiving praise can help to increase your intrinsic motivation. Praise yourself on a job well done and get your support team on board to give you praise and positive feedback on your progress.

If you already find a behaviour intrinsically rewarding don't add an extrinsic reward. Do it because you enjoy it. Research shows that giving an additional external reward for an already intrinsically rewarding behaviour can actually reduce your intrinsic motivation. An extrinsic reward can also have the effect of making something that you enjoy as fun or a hobby or 'play' feel like work. If you love reading about ancient civilisations because you find it fascinating, offering yourself a monetary reward for each chapter you read can actually reduce your enjoyment. It's worth noting that your intrinsic motivation won't be diluted if you happen to receive an external reward for engaging in a behaviour that you enjoy. If you decide, for example, to take your love of ancient civili-sation to the next level by studying it more formally in an online course, receiving a prize or an A+ won't affect your underlying motivation for learning about the subject. You'll just need to manage your expectation of future reward for your labour of love.

Believe that things will get better. Believe that you can beat brain fog by changing your habits. Believe that you will think faster, sharper, better. Believe that life will feel good again. Believe that you can reclaim your brain and find your 'self' again. Believe that you can shape an improved version of your 'self'. It won't be easy, but it won't take long and the reward will be worth the effort. In addition to effort, belief and determination you need a plan. That's where I come in.

30-day plan

Your 30-day plan begins with a planning day and ends with a final progress day, bookending four weeks spent building new habits to get you thinking faster, sharper, better. Each week has a different theme and rituals.

During week one, you will improve the quality of your sleep by making the 'Rise, Shine and Retire' rituals an integral part of your daily life. In week two, you will add the 'Smile' ritual to help you to better manage stress. The 'Challenge' and 'Nourish' rituals are added in weeks three and four, which focus on exercise and nutrition respectively. This approach allows you to layer the rituals into your life over the four weeks.

While each week has its own theme and rituals they are all interrelated and benefit all of the factors that affect brain fog. For example, some elements of the Retire ritual will help you to better manage stress, while some aspects of the 'Challenge' ritual will help you to sleep better. Good luck, and enjoy.

Planning day – day one

Yup, you guessed it! Today is all about planning.

1. Consult your intel

The intel that you have gleaned from your in-chapter assessments is invaluable and will help you to personalise your 30-day plan. Spend some time with this data today. Really look at it.

- Can you identify patterns or possible brain fog culprits?
- Make a note of unhealthy habits that need changing. .
- Identify cravings, triggers, routines and intrinsic and extrinsic rewards that you could harness to help you implement brain-healthy habits. As you now know, habits are most likely to stick if you sandwich your new routines between existing triggers and rewards.

2. Inform the troops

Successful habit change is more likely with good planning, self-knowledge and some support. Let your loved ones know that you are embarking on a 30-day journey to better brain health. Explain that you would like to block out a day when you can work on personalising your plan undisturbed but with their support if you need it.

3. Harness the power of routine

Daily rituals are powerful fog-busting routines that will change your life and get you thinking faster, sharper, better in just four weeks. Sticking to a regular schedule each day by embedding these six rituals in your daily routine will improve your brain function. It is really important to work with the natural rhythms of your body. If you are not a morning person, forcing yourself to exercise at 6 a.m. is a recipe for failure. Taking account of whether you are a lark or an owl, determine your ideal bedtime by working back from the time that you need to get up on most days. If you need to get up at 8 a.m. Monday to Friday, you need to follow that habit through on Saturdays and Sundays too. I know it seems tough, and it will be at first, but your brain will benefit immensely from the regularity and, before you know it, you will getting up at 8 a.m. every day without even thinking about it.

- Identify existing triggers and rewards that you could harness to help you to implement the daily rituals.
- Identify existing cravings that you could capitalise on to drive new healthy habits or list new cravings that you could cultivate.

4. Record your progress

In the first row of the table on the next page, rate your average sleep quality, stress levels, mood and energy over the last month. Then complete the table at the end of each of the four weeks. Keeping a record of your progress compared to your baseline will help to motivate you and keep you on track.

Sleep quality:

1= Slept soundly

2 = Slept well only woke for bathroom. Got back to sleep OK

3 = More than thirty minutes to fall asleep or woke more than twice

4 = Stayed awake more than twenty minutes after waking during the night

Stress levels:

1 = Stress levels off the scale

2 = A bit too stressed

3 = Hit my sweet spot

4 = Bored

Mood:

1 = Fantastic

2 = Good

3 = OK

4 = Low

Energy:

1 = Full of beans

2 = Good

3 = Tired

4 = Fatigued

Brain Fog Symptoms:

Use this column for comments you would like to note about your brain fog symptoms in the month prior to starting the 30-day plan.

General Comments:

Use this for any other comments you would like to note.

Day	Sleep	Stress	Mood	Energy	Brain Fog Symptoms	General Comments
Baseline on average						
Week 1						
Week 2						
Week 3						
Week 4						

Daily rituals

Regularity and repetition are key to creating brain-healthy habits. Before you start the programme, decide on the best time to carry out your rituals. If you deviate from the schedule, don't panic, just get yourself back on track as soon as you can. You have thirty days to turn these rituals into habits. The purpose of completing the table on the next page is to ensure that you optimise the timing of your daily rituals over the course of the next month, taking account of your natural rhythms, meals and existing commitments.

Routine	Best time
Wake	
Rise ritual	
Shine ritual	
Breakfast	
Lunch	
Dinner	
Exercise ritual	
Challenge ritual	
Smile ritual	
Retire ritual	
Go to bed	

The duration of specific rituals are suggested minimums; you can of course exercise for more than the recommended 150 minutes a week, laugh as much as you like or do several fun things every day if you wish. If you are already exercising for forty minutes a day, for example, keep that up, but for new routines I suggest that you start small. Once the routine becomes a habit you can build out from that solid base after you have completed the plan. The suggestions that I have included are not exhaustive, they are designed to get you started and to spark your imagination. You can also blend suggestions together – for example, smile while you do your thirty-minute workout or eat your brain-healthy lunch alfresco with friends who make you laugh. This is your plan, personalise it by doing the things that you love.

So many factors can contribute to brain fog and so many of those factors are intertwined it is likely that your brain fog is the result of multiple interacting factors. Your daily rituals will help you to build brain-healthy habits that will address many of these factors.

Focusing on something strengthens it. Try to focus on developing the new ritual rather than resisting old habits. Rehearse the new habit in your head. Simply imagining the new behaviour can help to build a new habit.

Adopting the daily rituals (Rise, Shine and Retire, Smile, Challenge and Nourish) will help you to beat brain fog. Don't worry, you don't have to adopt them all at once. Each week you will focus on one key aspect of your life that plays a critical role in how well your brain functions.

Week one – sleep

Without adequate sleep, you feel fatigued and your brain becomes sluggish and slow. The good news is that once you catch up on lost sleep and adopt good sleep hygiene you will sleep better, helping to clear your fog.

Your mission this week is to make sleep a priority every day by adopting the 'Rise, Shine and Retire' rituals which I've carefully designed to help you to sleep better. For the next seven days, focus your best efforts on going to bed and getting up at the same time and getting at least thirty minutes of daylight every single day. If you can achieve that you will have scored a major success and will notice a marked difference in your thinking.

Revisit the sleep assessment that you completed in Chapter 7. If you haven't already done so, have a look at whether you can remove any personal sleep disrupters which may be acting as barriers to sleep.

Sleep and stress are so intertwined that it is difficult to separate them. Managing stress is critical for sleep and sleep is fundamental to managing stress. As a consequence, certain elements of the Rise, Shine and Retire rituals will also help you to destress so that you will sleep better. This will provide a good foundation for week two, when you will focus on managing stress.

So, this week, concentrate on developing a regular sleep routine by going to bed and getting up at the same time every day, listening to your body and working with rather than against natural light. This will help you to synchronise your sleep–wake cycle with your natural rhythms and nature's rhythm of light and dark. Sweet dreams!

Week one: sleep rituals

RISE RITUAL

The Rise ritual takes less time than one snooze cycle on your phone. You can play around with the order until you find what works best for you – with one exception. Don't get out of bed until you smile.

1 Open your eyes

2 Smile (it's good to be alive)

3 Positive affirmation:

   o Sit on the side of your bed

   o As you place your feet on the ground, silently or aloud say, 'This is a good day' or any other positive affirmation

4 Go to the bathroom for a pee

5 Sixteen-second meditation

   o Breathe in for four, hold for four, breathe out for four and hold for four

6 Make your bed

7 Awaken your senses:

   o Open your sensory box (see page 194) and take out each item in turn, using your sense of smell, touch, sight, taste and sound

   o As you continue through your day, notice how the things that you encounter smell, feel, look, taste and sound

8 Stretch! You don't have to do a particular yoga sequence or a series of complicated exercises, just stretch your body in a way that feels good to you for five full minutes

Don't:

• Get out of bed until you smile!

• Reach for your phone

• Check emails or social media until you've completed your ritual and preferably, if you can manage it, not until you have eaten your breakfast

SHINE RITUAL

- Open curtains, shutters or blinds first thing in the morning

- Turn on a white light if it is dark outside

- Spend at least thirty minutes outside in daylight. As you progress through the four weeks, you can combine this with, for example, outdoor exercise, brain challenge, dining al fresco, meditation, etc. For now, the main thing is to get outside for at least thirty minutes, more if you can

- At 8 p.m., start to dim the lights around your house and make sure desaturation apps are activated on any screens you are using

- An hour before your scheduled bedtime, switch off all devices that emit blue light

- Close curtains, blinds and shutters and turn out all lights before you go to bed

RETIRE RITUAL

- Sixty to ninety minutes before your optimal bedtime:

  o Power off all of your devices and put them on charge

  o Perform your lock-up duties

  o Chat to your partner, kids, housemates, read a printed book or listen to an audiobook

- One hour before your optimal bedtime:

  o Turn off the heating (remember that a drop in temperature signals your body to sleep)

  o Brush your teeth, remove your make-up and complete any other bathroom activities

  o Change into your pyjamas

  o Write the following in your journal:

    - Any worries or 'to dos' running round your head

    - Something that you achieved today

    - Something that made you happy

- o Complete your progress record for the day
- Thirty minutes before bedtime:
  - o Engage in your chosen calming activity, such as:
    - – Listen to relaxing music
    - – Listen to a guided meditation
    - – Listen/watch an autonomous sensory meridian response (ASMR) video
    - – Meditate
    - – Take a warm bath or shower
    - – Light some candles
    - – Apply moisturiser to your body
    - – Get a foot massage from your partner or give yourself one

What one person finds calming another might find irritating. It is a very individual choice. The key is to find something that works for you.

- Five minutes before bedtime:
  - o Turn off the lights
  - o Get into bed

Week one: sleep rituals progress record

In the table below, enter the actual time that you completed the rituals each day. If you did not complete a ritual place an X in the box for that day. Make a note of anything that you think is pertinent: what worked, what didn't, how you felt, why you didn't complete a ritual, etc. You can

Week 1	Sleep	Wake time	Rise ritual
Mon	Time		
	Notes		
Tues	Time		
	Notes		
Weds	Time		
	Notes		
Thurs	Time		
	Notes		
Fri	Time		
	Notes		
Sat	Time		
	Notes		
Sun	Time		
	Notes		

use your bedside notebook to record more detail if you wish. Focus on the factors that influence your sleep. Record when you wake and when you go to bed. It's also helpful to estimate the time you fall asleep.

Shine ritual	Retire ritual	Bedtime	Asleep estimate

Week two – stress

If you are chronically stressed, it is practically impossible to think straight or stay focused. Making even the simplest of decisions can become overwhelming. You become forgetful, absent and find it tough to take in new information.

Your mission for week two is to smile, laugh, have fun and make a conscious effort to be in the moment. That doesn't sound too awful now, does it? Week two is about introducing and integrating effective stress-management behaviours into your daily routine so that they become second nature. Your brain will benefit and your fog will begin to clear if you stay present, laugh, smile and sleep regularly.

Getting regular restorative sleep is a brilliant first step towards managing stress. Continue with your Rise, Shine and Retire rituals, paying special attention to the stress-busting aspects. You can, of course, use the sixteen-second meditation throughout the day if you feel stress or anxiety rising.

If you are currently chronically stressed, take remedial action by putting some extra work into getting your stress system back in balance. You can do this through self-talk by consciously activating your thinking brain, getting it to talk to your emotional brain and coax your amygdala down from the ledge of high alertness and irrational, unnecessary, constant fear.

Reread Chapter 2 if you feel you need to and take some time to do the following:

- Declutter your brain
- Declutter your surroundings
- Get organised
- Remove distractions
- Seek support
- Set aside some time to work through what is stressing you
- Seek professional help if necessary

Set a specific time once a week or once a day depending on your needs to deal with your chronic stress.

Aoife, who has multiple sclerosis, explained to me that when she was first diagnosed all she could think of was her MS and all the dreadful things that might happen to her body, her brain and her life if the disease progresses. She was consumed by it. After attending one of my talks, she decided that she would do her MS worrying on Tuesday afternoons between 3 p.m. and 4 p.m. If a worry popped into her head she wrote it down or made a mental note to revisit it at 3 p.m. on Tuesday. You can do something similar. During your designated hour, write down your worries. Get a clear picture of what is stressing you and why. Then ask yourself what you can and can't do about them. If there is nothing you can do then work on accepting them. If there is something you can do then devise a realistic plan and implement it.

There is an old Irish proverb that says, 'A laugh and a long sleep are the two best cures for anything.' I love when neuroscience backs up old words of wisdom.

Week two: stress rituals

'SMILE' RITUAL

The aim of this ritual is to smile more and stress less. Smiling and laughter not only reduce stress, they also boost immune function. Focusing on the present will improve your attentional capacity and help you to manage stress effectively. If it feels like it's been a long time since you've smiled, laughed or had fun, or you feel that you've lost your connection with your fun side, don't worry – it happens to all of us from time to time especially when we are stressed. But smiling, laughing and having fun are simply choices that we make. If we consciously and actively make those choices every day, with time, smiling, laughing and having fun will become habits. Act the way you want to feel and soon you will feel the way that you want.

- Smile:
  - o When you wake
  - o When you pee
  - o When you shower
  - o When you look in the mirror
  - o When you put the kettle on

- o When you sit down to eat
- o When you greet another human
- o When you exercise
- Find at least one thing to laugh about every day
- Do at least one fun thing every day
- Be present in the moment

Smile more, stress less suggestions

- Schedule a pleasant event, do something that makes you feel special
- Place some Post-it notes with fun quotes or jokes on your fridge, laptop and/or mirror
- Start collecting funny jokes, cartoons, memes or videos that make you laugh in a folder on your computer or physically in a notebook or box. Then you will have a stash to return to time and again if you need a reason to laugh, or better still, share them with someone else. Smiling is contagious – their smile may spark yours
- Pick one fun thing that you usually feel too tired to do and do it anyway
- Do something that you loved doing as a child (yes, you can splash in puddles)
- Dance like no one is watching
- Put on funny voices
- Spend time in the company of people who make you laugh
- Laugh out loud at your child's knock, knock, jokes even if they're not funny and you've heard them a million times
- Watch a funny movie
- Listen to a comedy podcast
- Watch your favourite episode of *Friends*
- Pick up an item from your living room and look at it, really look at it; notice its weight, texture and smell

- Close your eyes for thirty seconds and count how many sounds you can hear
- Focus on your surroundings, on what can you see or hear, take notice of what the seat or ground feels like underneath you
- Learn a joke a day
- Tell a joke a day
- Try to see beauty in the world around you – you'll be surprised how you can find beauty in the mundane if you decide to look
- Be present when you engage in your daily rituals
- Take a moment to focus on your breath
- Play with your kids and/or your dog or cat, or tell your budgie jokes

Week two: stress rituals progress record

During week two, keep a record of the following in the table below:

Smile: Record the number of times you smiled today, noting how it made you feel.

Contagion: Record the number of smiles you induce by sharing your smile.

Laughter: Record the number of times you laughed and why.

Fun: Detail the fun activity that you intentionally chose to do today. Also check in with yourself throughout the day and note any time you find yourself having fun by accident.

Week 2	Stress	Smile	Contagion	
Mon	Frequency: Activity: Notes:			
Tues	Frequency: Activity: Notes:			
Weds	Frequency: Activity: Notes:			
Thurs	Frequency: Activity: Notes:			
Fri	Frequency: Activity: Notes:			
Sat	Frequency: Activity: Notes:			
Sun	Frequency: Activity: Notes:			

Present: Detail the activity that you devoted your full, undivided attention to today. Note how being fully present, engaged in what you were doing while you were doing it, made you feel.

Other: Make a note of any other actions that you took or eradicated to help you to better manage stress.

In addition, continue to keep a record of your sleep rituals in the table below.

Laughter	Fun	Present	Other

Week 2	Sleep	Wake time	Rise ritual	
Mon	Time			
	Notes			
Tues	Time			
	Notes			
Weds	Time			
	Notes			
Thurs	Time			
	Notes			
Fri	Time			
	Notes			
Sat	Time			
	Notes			
Sun	Time			
	Notes			

Shine ritual	Retire ritual	Bedtime	Asleep estimate

Week three – exercise

Without challenge, your brain will shrink with each passing year and your brain function will suffer. Without physical exercise, you compromise your cardiovascular system – the very system that your brain depends upon for vital oxygen and energy. Challenging your brain and exercising your body regularly will help to ensure that your brain has sufficient resources and adequate oxygen and nutrients to think faster, sharper, better.

Your mission for week three is to focus your best efforts on exercising your brain and your body. You need to add physically and mentally challenging rituals to your day while you continue with your sleep and stress rituals. Take a moment to acknowledge the progress that you have made in weeks one and two.

If you struggle with getting regular exercise or find that you don't want to exercise, look back at the work that you did on triggers and rewards on your planning day and don't forget to cultivate a craving for exercise. Now would be a good time to reread Chapter 9 for practical tips to help you to optimise your chances of success. Any exercise for your brain and for your body is better than none.

Make sure that you take your natural rhythms into account. Simply switching the time that you exercise to later or earlier in the day when you feel more alert might make a big difference. You can also use this as an opportunity to tweak the timing of your rituals from week one and two.

If you find it difficult to establish an exercise habit, it could simply be that you are doing a physical activity that you don't enjoy. Look for fun things you can do that involve exercise. Think outside the box. Add a competitive element. Maybe you need the motivation of exercising with others, group classes, a personal trainer or playing a team sport.

When it comes to challenging your brain, it is critical to choose something that you love. If you are finding that you don't want to challenge your brain, see whether you can tease apart why that is. Could it be that you have some old hang-ups from your school days about learning? Perhaps you are anxious about trying new things. Addressing the underlying issue should help you to make progress. Challenging your brain and learning new things should be fun – by definition it will be challenging but that doesn't mean it can't be enjoyable and learning is rewarding.

Physical exercise and brain challenges can be integrated into other aspects of your life, they don't have to be stand alone. As you work through the programme, many daily rituals will allow you to tick more than one box because they overlap. For example, engaging in a team sport that you find fun can provide opportunity for de-stressing laughter, the exercise will help you to sleep and, depending on the nature of the sport, it may also provide you with a cognitive challenge.

Don't limit your challenges, challenge your limits. Physical activity where the level of offort required matches your level of fitness is generally safe for everyone, at any age. People who are physically fit have less chance of injury than those who are not fit. Always exercise safely and seek the advice of your doctor before taking on a new exercise regime, especially if you:

- are over fifty and are not used to energetic activity.
- have a diagnosed chronic condition such as diabetes, heart dis-ease or osteoarthritis.
- have symptoms such as chest pain or pressure, dizziness or joint pain.

If chronic illness, mobility issues or a degenerative condition prevent you from doing the recommended amount of physical activity, be as active as you are able to be. And be imaginative – for example, could drumming work? Do some research or ask members of your medical team for suggestions so that you can exercise safely within the constraints of your condition. Start slowly and build your level of activity over time, particularly if you haven't been active for a long while.

Week three: exercise rituals

EXERCISE RITUAL

The critical thing to remember about exercising both your brain and your body is to acknowledge your current baseline and aim for progress in small, achievable increments. Set realistic goals and track your progress incrementally from your baseline rather than measuring the distance from your goal. It's not helpful if you've never jogged before to compare yourself to someone who runs 10k a day. If you've never run before, running for ten minutes a day is a massive achievement that your brain will benefit from. Remember your goal to clear that damn fog is far more important than running marathons or joining Mensa.

The good news is that both physical and mental exercise will help you to boost brain function and beat brain fog. A life filled with novelty and challenge has the added bonus of increasing your happiness levels.

Challenge your brain

- Engage in mentally stimulating activities that challenge your brain for thirty minutes on at least five days (see below for suggestions)

- Try something new every day – take a new route to work, go to a new coffee shop, try a different food

- Learn something every day

- Choose a time of day when you feel most mentally alert for your challenge activity:
  - o Early morning
  - o Mid-morning
  - o Lunchtime
  - o Mid-afternoon
  - o Early evening

Exercise your brain suggestions

- Challenge yourself to learn how to:
  - o Skateboard

- o Knit a scarf
- o Draw a portrait
- o Sew a button on a shirt
- o Make a dress
- o Swim
- o Line dance
- o Speak Spanish
- o Restore cars
- o Apply make-up like a pro
- o Give your hair the latest curls or waves
- o Use a new app
- o Use Excel
- o Write code
- o Garden
- o Cook
- o Bake
- o Choose your own activity – the possibilities are endless
- Do something creative:
  - o Make an artistic picture with pen, pencil, paints or your phone
  - o Write a poem, short story, song, lyric or limerick
  - o Arrange some flowers
  - o Read photography tips and techniques to improve your phone photography skills
- Learn a new fact today and pass it on to someone together with the reason they need to know it
- If you already do puzzles, challenge yourself to move to a harder level or complete your regular level in a shorter period of time
- Play a strategy game like chess
- Learn about something or someone from a different culture, ethnicity or background

- Visit a museum, art gallery, historical building or exhibition
- Read a poem or song lyric and try to interpret its meaning
- Memorise the words of a song, poem, speech or quote
- Memorise the stops on your commute and try to recall them on the journey home
- Memorise the names of the parents at your kid's school
- Read a section of the newspaper you wouldn't normally read
- Tune in to a difference radio station
- Listen to a different genre of music
- Read a book from a genre you wouldn't normally read
- Join a book club with friends or online to discuss and critically analyse what you read
- Have a conversation with someone you've never spoken to before
- Try something outside your comfort zone
- Try a new vegetable
- Try a new restaurant
- Try a new recipe
- Try a food you've never tasted before
- Order something different from the menu at your favourite restaurant
- Sort your clothes according to colour, type or frequency of use
- Do something, anything that you have never done before
- Do something out of the ordinary at lunchtime
- Go somewhere in easy reach of your home or workplace that you've never been to before
- Try walking a new route to work
- Change your jogging route
- Take up a new sport or try a new technique
- Start, plan and execute a home improvement or gardening project

- Learn the names of the plants in your garden
- Make greeting cards

I also encourage you to take a long-term approach to challenging your brain on an ongoing basis. I have included some options for you to consider:

- Reignite your curiosity:
  - Make a list of things that have always fascinated you and promise to learn more about them
  - Diversify your interests
  - Become curious about other cultures, viewpoints and world views
- Embrace education:
  - Check out evening classes to see if there is anything that takes your fancy
  - Sign up for a free Massive Open Online Course
  - Study for a qualification, diploma or degree in a subject that fascinates you
- Take your hobby to the next level:
  - Resume a long forgotten hobby
  - Take up a new hobby
  - Take a current passion to the next level

Exercise your body

- The recommended guidelines are to do at least 150 minutes of moderate intensity activity (e.g. riding a bike, brisk walking or pushing a lawnmower) a week or 75 minutes of vigorous intensity activity (jogging, running, riding a bike fast or uphill, walking upstairs, playing football, rugby, netball, etc.) a week. You can achieve this weekly target in multiple ways. For example, you can do several short sessions of vigorous activity; you can mix moderate and vigorous sessions over two or more days or, if you prefer, you can reach your weekly target on one day. Having said that, I would recommend that you try to do some form of physical activity every day. Even five minutes is better than nothing

- Remember you can incorporate exercise into your daily routine; for example, by walking to work or the gym, by taking the stairs instead of the lift or by doing heavy housework or gardening

- It is important to include strength training or weight-bearing exercise on at least two days per week. Consider working on alternating major muscle groups on different days; for example, legs, hips and back one day and abdomen, chest, shoulders and arms on another

- Break up long periods of inactivity and reduce the amount of time you spend sitting or lying down

- Try to incorporate balance exercises each week. For example, try standing on one foot; as your balance improves, you can try holding the non-weight-bearing leg out to the side or behind you (don't forget to alternate legs). Walk heel-to-toe in a straight line as if you were walking along a tightrope or stand up and sit down on a chair without using your hands

- Choose a time of day for your main blocks of exercise that works best for you

Week three: exercise rituals progress record

During week three, along with your sleep and stress rituals, keep a record of the following in the table on the next page:

Challenge: Record the number of minutes you spent engaging in your chosen brain challenge. Describe the challenge and note how your feel.

Change: Note any new experiences you have – it can be something really simple like eating a vegetable you never tasted before, smelling a new scent, turning the dial to a new radio station or changing the route that you walk to work.

Learn: Record something new that you learned today.

Aerobic: Note the intensity and duration of any aerobic activity you engage in and make a note of any exercise that you integrated into your daily routine.

Resistance: Note the type and duration of any resistance training that you engaged in.

Stand: Estimate how much time you spent sitting and how much time you spent standing and note the how often you completed balance exercises.

Week 3	Exercise	Challenge	Change
Mon	Duration: Activity: Notes:		
Tues	Duration: Activity: Notes:		
Weds	Duration: Activity: Notes:		
Thurs	Duration: Activity: Notes:		
Fri	Duration: Activity: Notes:		
Sat	Duration: Activity: Notes:		
Sun	Duration: Activity: Notes:		

Learn	Aerobic	Resistance	Stand

Week 3	Stress	Smile	Contagion
Mon	Frequency: Activity: Notes:		
Tues	Frequency: Activity: Notes:		
Weds	Frequency: Activity: Notes:		
Thurs	Frequency: Activity: Notes:		
Fri	Frequency: Activity: Notes:		
Sat	Frequency: Activity: Notes:		
Sun	Frequency: Activity: Notes:		

Laughter	Fun	Present	Other

Week 3	Sleep	Wake time	Rise Ritual
Mon	Time		
	Notes		
Tues	Time		
	Notes		
Weds	Time		
	Notes		
Thurs	Time		
	Notes		
Fri	Time		
	Notes		
Sat	Time		
	Notes		
Sun	Time		
	Notes		

Shine Ritual	Retire Ritual	Bedtime	Asleep estimate

Week four – nutrition

Your brain is at your mercy. If you give it any old rubbish to eat then don't be surprised if what it produces is rubbish too. Treat your brain, and yourself, with respect by eating brain-healthy meals. Your mission for week four is to focus your best efforts on following a delicious and uncomplicated Mediterranean diet. Commit to consuming only fresh, healthy food from now on. After all, you are worth it. Eat consciously and think of every meal as an opportunity to nourish your brain.

By now your sleep and stress rituals should be feeling less effortful and you may even be starting to enjoy exercises and challenge. Even if you're not yet, keep exercising your body and challenging your brain as good results are just around the corner.

Week four: nutrition ritual

NOURISH RITUAL

The aim of this ritual is to ensure that your brain receives the nourishment it needs at the right time so that it can maintain homeostasis and perform to its optimum level, helping you to think faster, sharper, better. The best way to do this is to eat at regular times and follow a Mediterranean diet rich in foods that reduce inflammation, oxidative stress and insulin resistance. The diet is pretty straightforward to follow and there is no reason why you can't switch to it immediately. At the end of this chapter, you'll find a few of my favourite recipes. I've listed some small changes that you can make to your existing diet if you would prefer to adopt a more gradual approach to switching to a Mediterranean diet. Having protein (e.g. fish or poultry, or small amounts of lean meat, eggs, cheese, beans, nuts) with every meal will stabilise your energy levels and help you to stay alert throughout the day. Keep protein portions under 100 grams.

To complete your Nourish Ritual:

- Eat breakfast at the same time every morning:

  - A brain-healthy breakfast should contain both protein and antioxidants (e.g. fruits and vegetables such as blueberries, apples, broccoli and spinach)

- Eat lunch at the same time every day:

  o Avoid sandwiches and pre-packaged food high in preservatives

  o Consider homemade soup, a colourful salad or mixed platters (veggies, fruits, fresh seafood and/or poultry, for example)

- Eat dinner at the same time every day:

  o Try to finish eating at least two to three hours before lying down to sleep. This will give time for digestion and help you to avoid reflux, which can interfere with sleep. Research shows that eating dinner at 10 p.m. increases cortisol and blood sugars as well as reduces fat burning, compared to eating dinner at 6 p.m.

  o Aim for a dinner of lean protein and lots of vegetables

  o If you've missed dinner or need to eat late opt for calming foods like lean proteins (e.g. turkey, chicken or fish) that boost serotonin and help you to feel sleepy. Alternatively, combine these foods with complex carbohydrates such as whole wheat crackers or brown rice an hour before bedtime. Shredding a few basil leaves or eating some walnuts, almonds or cashews will also boost serotonin and help you to relax

- If you wish to snack, consider healthy options like berries, avocado toast, roasted pumpkin seeds, sunflower seeds, sliced peppers or carrots with hummus and nuts (though avoid salted nuts)

Diet Dos

- Follow a Mediterranean diet that fights inflammation, oxidative stress and insulin resistance

- Eat plenty of green leafy vegetables

- Eat plenty of colourful fruit and vegetables, legumes, beans, whole grains, nuts, seeds and lean high-quality protein

- Eat foods high in omega-3 (e.g. salmon, tuna, dark leafy vegetables, flax oil, flax seed)

- Eat anti-inflammatory foods (e.g. blueberries, red and purple berries and grapes, apples, broccoli, kale, tomatoes, yellow onions and scallions, leafy vegetables, oily fish, flax seed and flax oil)

- Eat foods containing vitamin D (e.g. salmon, tuna, sole, eggs, fortified cereals and milk)

- Use olive oil as your main source of fat

- Drink plenty of water

- Share meals with other people. Eating is not just about nutrition, it is a social event and an opportunity to stimulate your brain and have fun through conversation and laughter

Some small changes that you can make one day at a time, if you are taking a more gradual approach:

- Have a day free from processed food

- Read the food labels today, pay attention to the sodium content

- Have a snack-free day

- Have a sugar-free day, read the labels

- Try not to eat after 7 p.m. today

- If you are overweight, reduce your portions by 10 per cent today

- Drink a healthy amount of fluids based on your BMI

- Eat a portion of brightly coloured fruit today

- Eat a portion of dark green vegetables today

- Spend more time cooking than eating today

- Substitute a regular snack with a low-sugar fruit snack today (e.g. berries)

- Read the labels on all the food you consume today

- Have a chocolate-free day today

- Prepare at least one healthy meal from fresh ingredients today

- Have an alcohol-free day today

Diet Don'ts

- Don't eat processed foods, such as ready meals, microwave meals, savoury snacks, crisps, pies, pasties, cakes, biscuits, processed meats

- Don't take supplements unless you have been prescribed them by your doctor to address a diagnosed deficiency

- Don't eat foods with high salt content such as smoked, salted or cured meat or fish (i.e. bacon, sausages, sardines), frozen dinners, salted nuts, processed cheeses, shop bought-sauces, pizza, croutons, salted crackers, canned and dehydrated soups

- Don't consume foods or drinks high in sugar, such as sweets, cakes, chocolate and biscuits. In addition, watch out for foods that you might otherwise consider healthy or savoury such as fruit juices, canned fruit in its own juice, granola, protein bars, low-fat products including yoghurt, premade pasta sauces, processed soups, ketchup, cereals and cereal bars. Check the label as they could be unexpected sources of sugar, or even have had sugar added to enhance the flavour

- Don't snack after dinner

- Don't eat red meat (beef, lamb, pork, veal, venison, etc.) and processed meats such as salami, bacon, sausages, pepperoni, deli meats including processed turkey and ham. Slices from turkey roasted in the store are fine

- Don't eat refined grains such as white bread and pasta

- Don't eat saturated fats which are found in things like pastries and pies, fatty meat (i.e. lamb), processed meats, full-fat dairy products (i.e. milk, yogurt, cheese), white chocolate, toffee, cakes, biscuits

- Don't drink alcohol at all, if you can avoid it. If you can't, then:

  o Avoid alcohol after 8 p.m.

  o Have several alcohol-free days each week

Week four: nutrition rituals progress record

During week four, using the table on the next page, keep a record of the times at which you eat breakfast, lunch and dinner. Also keep a note of what you eat at each meal and any snacks that you have. Note how you feel after each meal, with a specific focus on your brain fog symptoms, mood and alertness levels, as this will help you to identify any potential trigger foods.

Week 4	Breakfast	Lunch	Dinner	
Mon Time: Food: Notes:				
Tues Time: Food: Notes:				
Weds Time: Food: Notes:				
Thurs Time: Food: Notes:				
Fri Time: Food: Notes:				
Sat Time: Food: Notes:				
Sun Time: Food: Notes:				

Snacks	Brain fog	Alertness	Mood

Continue to keep a record of your sleep, stress and exercise rituals in the table below.

Week 4	Exercise	Challenge	Change
Mon	Duration: Activity: Notes:		
Tues	Duration: Activity: Notes:		
Weds	Duration: Activity: Notes:		
Thurs	Duration: Activity: Notes:		
Fri	Duration: Activity: Notes:		
Sat	Duration: Activity: Notes:		
Sun	Duration: Activity: Notes:		

Learn	Aerobic	Resistance	Stand

Week 4	Stress	Smile	Contagion
Mon	Frequency: Activity: Notes:		
Tues	Frequency: Activity: Notes:		
Weds	Frequency: Activity: Notes:		
Thurs	Frequency: Activity: Notes:		
Fri	Frequency: Activity: Notes:		
Sat	Frequency: Activity: Notes:		
Sun	Frequency: Activity: Notes:		

Laughter	Fun	Present	Other

Week 4	Sleep	Wake time	Rise ritual
Mon	Time		
	Notes		
Tues	Time		
	Notes		
Weds	Time		
	Notes		
Thurs	Time		
	Notes		
Fri	Time		
	Notes		
Sat	Time		
	Notes		
Sun	Time		
	Notes		

Shine ritual	Retire ritual	Bedtime	Asleep estimate

My personal daily rituals

It is so important to personalise your plan, to do things that you love or have meaning for you at the times that work best for you. I thought it might be useful to share some of my daily rituals with you. I mainly work from home, writing or podcasting, but when I have to travel or have work commitments outside my home I adjust my rituals accordingly.

I don't beat myself up if I have 'off' days – I consider that listening to my body. If I have a flare-up, feel fatigue, pain or brain fog, which thankfully only occur occasionally, I pay attention to what my body is telling me and take restorative action sooner rather than later. In recent years, my symptoms are generally mild but they are still significant enough to remind me that I used to live in constant pain, always fatigued and foggy. I take it as a warning sign that something is amiss and a signal to take some time out, slow down a little and reset.

When I take stock at such times, I realise that I may have slipped back into overworking, often as a consequence of letting my stress levels slide beyond my sweet spot. I give my body some time to recover and then I get myself back on track with my daily rituals as soon as I can. I know deep down that these daily rituals are the healthy habits that keep me energised and able to think faster, sharper, better.

As soon as I open my eyes in the morning I make a big smiley face. I suspect that I look a little crazy but I don't care. Honestly, I can't tell you how much benefit this first smile brings me. It sets me up for the day. I feel good before I'm even fully awake and, importantly, before I have had time to decide otherwise.

I swing my legs to the side of the bed and, as my feet touch the ground, I say to myself, 'This is a good day.' I do my sixteen-second meditation (box breathing) while I open the bedroom shutters. I go out to the garden to feed the birds. I like to watch them feed while I have breakfast. My default is to spend a lot of time inside my head, thinking, planning, working, and so it is good for me to start the day by looking outside myself. I feel fully present in the moment and connected with the world around me when I feed the birds and take a little wander around my garden, looking at new buds and deadheading.

My brain is sharpest and most creative in the early morning. I like to rise early. Getting three or four hours of writing under my belt by 11 a.m.

appeases the 'to-do' master in my brain enough to allow me to pause to get my exercise in before lunch. My brain usually needs a break at this point and I find that the exercise clears my head and refreshes my brain. I alternate between walking, cycling or lifting weights in the gym.

I am ravenous after exercise so I tuck into delicious homemade soup or tuna salad. My husband, Dave, and I try to make all of our meals from scratch using fresh ingredients – I've included some of my favourite brain-healthy recipes below; they are packed with goodness and easy to make.

In the afternoon, I work in a different room. I find that the change of scenery makes it feel like starting a new day rather than heading into an afternoon slump. However, if I do feel my alertness dropping around 2 or 3 p.m. I'll close my eyes for 10 minutes. Wherever I work, I always have something tactile like an soft faux-fur throw or a velvet cushion close to hand. I also like to light an aromatherapy candle. I find the scent and having something soft to touch very calming. It makes working more pleasant and less stressful. Taking short breaks to cuddle and play with my dogs, who always make me smile, is another great stress buster.

Dave and I make a point of eating our evening meal together. It's an important ritual for us and something we always did as a family when the kids lived at home. It's an opportunity for us to catch up, share news or offload. It's also good for me to exercise my social skills, especially as I spend so much time in my head working alone.

Evenings are generally very chilled. I'm not one for pubs or big nights out and I rarely watch TV. After dinner I like to get into my pyjamas, turn off the overhead lights and read on the sofa by lamplight with my dogs snuggled beside me. Around 11 p.m. I climb the stairs with a glass of water. I close the shutters and the door and turn off the lights to make the room as dark and as quiet as possible.

Brain-healthy recipes

At-a-glance guide to brain-healthy eating

Essential	Optional	Limit or Exclude
Berries	Beans and Legumes	Added sugar
Fish	Eggs	Cakes and pastries
Healthy fats (e.g. olive oil)	Fruits	Fried food
Nuts	Grains (preferably wholegrain)	Processed food
Vegetables (especially green leafy or brightly coloured varieties)	Poultry	Red meat (including sausages, deli meats, luncheon meats, salamis, ham, bacon etc.)
	Dairy (e.g. yogurt, milk)	
	Sea salt	Table salt

Breakfasts

BERRY SMOOTHIE

Brain health benefits

Berries are rich in antioxidants that reduce inflammation and oxidative stress. Antioxidants are a great weapon in the fight against brain fog because they can improve communication between brain cells and support memory by boosting the brain's ability to grow new connections (neuroplasticity). They also help prevent inflammation and may reduce risk of age-related cognitive decline. They may even give your mood a lift.

Almond milk is high in vitamin E, which is both an antioxidant and a good alternative to full-fat milk because it is rich in healthy fats. Almond milk will help you to feel fuller for longer.

Ingredients

Serves 2

> *250g fresh or frozen berries (e.g. blackberries, blackcurrants, blueberries, raspberries, strawberries – I like a mix, but you may wish to stick to one kind)*
> *250g low-fat or fat-free yogurt – any flavour, I like raspberry*
> *100ml unsweetened almond milk*
> *Optional: 25g of porridge oats or a tablespoon of chia seeds*

Method

Whizz all of the ingredients in a blender until smooth. That's it, couldn't be simpler! Using frozen berries will produce a thicker smoothie. If you are using fresh berries but would like a thicker consistency, add some banana or ice.

WARM HARD-BOILED EGG SALAD

Brain health benefits

While there is no research directly linking eating eggs to better brain health, there is considerable evidence demonstrating a link between better brain function and the nutrients found in eggs, including B vitamins and choline, a micronutrient involved in the production of a neurotransmitter that helps to regulate mood and memory.

Onions are a great source of B vitamins and tomatoes have antioxidant properties, while cucumber contains a particular antioxidant called fisetin which may enhance memory.

Ingredients

Serves 1

2 medium to large eggs
4 cherry tomatoes, roughly chopped
2.5cm of cucumber, skin removed and finely diced
A few rings of red onion, finely diced
1 tsp of butter

Method

Bring a pot of water to the boil. Using a slotted spoon, add two eggs to the water. Leave the eggs to boil for eleven minutes. While the eggs are boiling, chop up some cherry tomatoes, skinned cucumber and red onion into really small pieces.

Remove the shell from the eggs and roughly chop them into a serving bowl. Add a small knob of butter and mash into the egg as it melts. Thoroughly mix the salad ingredients through the egg mix. A tiny twist of sea salt or pepper can bring the flavours out.

Lunches

ROASTED TOMATO, PEPPER AND GARLIC SOUP

Brain health benefits

Tomatoes are a source of a powerful antioxidant, called lycopene, which helps to defend the brain from free-radical damage. Red peppers are an excellent source of vitamin B6, which helps the body to produce hormones including noradrenaline and melatonin.

Ingredients

Serves 4

350g tomatoes, any kind
300g deseeded red and/or yellow peppers
6 cloves of garlic
Extra virgin olive oil for brushing
400ml low-salt vegetable or chicken stock
300ml low-fat milk
Freshly ground black pepper
Optional: fresh chilli (deseeded) or chilli flakes

Method

Pre-heat oven to 200°C. Slice large tomatoes or cut cherry tomatoes in half. Cut the peppers into quarters or sixths. Remove the skin from the garlic cloves. Place the tomatoes, peppers, garlic and fresh chilli (if using) into a roasting dish, lightly brushing them with a small amount of extra virgin olive oil. Season with freshly ground black pepper. Place in the oven to roast for twenty-five to thirty minutes, although check them after twenty minutes to avoid charring. If you are using a soup maker, transfer the vegetables, add stock and milk, set to smooth and about twenty minutes later you will have delicious, smooth soup. Alternatively, transfer the vegetables to a deep pan or pot, add the stock and the milk and simmer for twenty-five minutes with no lid. Transfer to a blender and blend till smooth.

FRENCH ONION SOUP

Brain health benefits

Onions are bursting with flavour and packed with nutrients – in fact, they are one of nature's best sources of B vitamins. The folate in B vitamins is particularly good at clearing up debris that can build up and increase the risk of stroke and dementia.

Ingredients

Serves 4

3 medium white onions, peeled
2 medium red onions, peeled
6 cloves of garlic
Extra-virgin olive oil
1 litre low-salt vegetable stock made with two stock cubes

Method

Slice the onions and crush the garlic cloves. Heat the olive oil in a deep fying pan and add the garlic and onions. Cook over a low heat for approximately ten minutes, without stirring the onions too much. Essentially you need to wait until the onions cook down to the point where their sugars start to caramelise and turn brown. The darker the onions become, the sweeter the soup. I don't like my soup too sweet so I turn the heat off when the onions are lightly browned.

Transfer the onions to a soup maker, add the stock, select smooth and wait twenty-one minutes (well, that's how long it takes in my soup maker). If you don't have a soup maker, add the stock to the pan, cover and simmer for twenty-five minutes. Blend in the pot using a hand blender or transfer to a blonder.

Tip: a small portion of caramelised onions make a tasty topping for other meals including healthy turkey burgers.

Dinners

SALMON PESTO WITH ALMOND CRUST WITH CABBAGE AND BROCCOLI

This tasty salmon dish is a great way to get omega-3 into your diet. Aim to eat at least two 100g servings of fatty fish each week. Other fatty fish rich in omega-3 include cod, mackerel, herring and light tuna. Omega-3 plays an important role in the maintaining brain cell health.

The tasty almond crust will also benefit your brain because almonds are packed with vitamins and minerals. Almonds are one of the best sources of vitamin E, which is an antioxidant. Research suggests that healthy levels of vitamin E may boost alertness and prevent decline in cognitive function.

Pine nuts, a key ingredient of pesto, are rich in zinc, known to benefit hormonal health. In addition to a high antioxidant content, they are a good source of healthy fats, fibre, vitamins and minerals. They also contain iron, which is important for the transportation of oxygen throughout your body and brain. As an added bonus, unsaturated fats in pine nuts increase insulin sensitivity, which is good news for diabetics.

Cabbage is low in calories and high in nutrients, including: vitamin B6, which is essential for energy metabolism and normal functioning of the nervous system, and antioxidants to protect from free-radical damage. Broccoli is a good source of cognition-enhancing vitamin K and also has both antioxidant and anti-inflammatory properties.

However, you can go for any green leafy vegetables with this dish; most are rich in brain-healthy nutrients and antioxidants, including vitamin E, vitamin K, folate and beta carotene.

Ingredients

Serves 2

2 salmon fillet steaks
Enough olive oil to grease the baking tray
Half a lemon
Black pepper to taste
2 level tbsp fresh basil pesto
2 level tbsp finely ground almonds
1 level tbsp freshly grated parmesan cheese
Cabbage heart, sliced thinly
Broccoli

Method

Preheat your oven to 230°C. Cover a baking tray with tin foil and lightly grease with olive oil. Run your hand gently around the fish to remove any bones that were missed during filleting. Leave the skin on the fish. Place the fillets skin-side down on the baking tray. Squeeze lemon over both fillets and season with pepper.

Place all of the pesto in a small bowl. Mix a third of the almonds with the pesto, giving it a good stir to form a paste. Spread the paste evenly over the top of the two salmon fillets. Mix half of the parmesan with the remaining almonds and spread over the paste. Scatter the remaining parmesan over the two fillets. Place in the middle shelf of the oven and cook for ten minutes. The crust should be crispy and the salmon fillets should be moist.

While the salmon is cooking, wash and trim the cabbage and broccoli and steam for five minutes. When tender, add a squeeze of lemon and serve hot with the salmon fillets.

GARLIC CHICKEN WITH ROAST SWEET POTATO FRIES

Brain health benefits

Skinless chicken is a great source of lean protein. It is a good source of B vitamins, which are neuroprotective, and choline, which is a building block of acetylcholine, a neurotransmitter, that helps memory function. Tomatoes are rich in lycopene, which may boost learning and memory.

Sweet potatoes are highly nutritious and contain beta carotene. Low levels of beta carotene have been associated with poor cognitive function.

Ingredients

Serves 4

4 lean chicken fillets
1 litre of low-salt chicken stock
6 juicy sun-dried tomatoes
6 cloves of garlic, peeled, crushed
1 small chilli
1 tbsp tomato puree
4 medium-sized sweet potatoes
1 tbsp olive oil
Paprika, black and red pepper or Cajun seasoning

Method

Pre-heat the oven to 200°C. Slice the chicken fillets lengthways into strips about the size of a goujon. Lay them in an open casserole or ceramic oven dish. Pour the stock over the chicken. Add the sun-dried tomatoes, garlic, chilli and tomato puree and stir gently till mixed. Place in the oven and cook for forty minutes.

Peel and wash the sweet potatoes, slice into chip slices according to your own preference – chunky or slender. Place the sliced sweet potatoes in an oven tray, add some olive oil and the seasoning of your choosing – paprika, black and red pepper or Cajun seasoning. Mix with your hands till the fries are well coated. Place on the middle shelf of the oven and cook for 25 to 35 minutes and serve with the garlic chicken.

Snacks

Ditch processed and packaged snacks and sweets for the brain-healthy options below.

Berries

Satisfy your sweet tooth and sugar cravings with berries rich in antioxidants that reduce inflammation and oxidative stress. Replace a bag of sweets with a handful any of the following: blackberries, blackcurrants, blueberries, raspberries or strawberries.

Nuts and seeds

Replace crisps, chips and other snacks that satisfy your crunchy craving with a handful of nuts and seeds. Walnuts, almonds, pecans, hazelnuts, pumpkin seeds, sunflower seeds – the options are almost endless but go for raw and unsalted.

Nuts are excellent sources of protein and a good source of omega-3, which is good for brain cell health. They are also packed with vitamin E, which has brain-protective properties. Now I know you might be thinking that snacking on nuts could lead to weight gain due to their high calorie content. However, research says that they can actually aid weight loss by helping you to feel fuller for longer. Nonetheless, don't overindulge and avoid salted or dry roasted packaged nuts. Remember, peanuts are a legume, not a nut.

Progress day: day 30

Take today to celebrate your successes and enjoy the progress that you have made. I also want you to take some time to look at what worked and what didn't, so that you can make some adjustments going forward. Remember this is only the start of your fog-free journey; you need to keep on doing what you are doing, but you must never be satisfied with that because your brain needs to be challenged to thrive. Congratulate yourself but avoid complacency.

Use the box below to update your brain fog profile and compare it to the brain fog profile that you completed in Chapter 1.

Indicate the domains in which you experienced symptoms over the thirty days. On a scale of one to five, indicate how frequently you experience these symptoms.

1 = infrequently (less than once a month – or not in the last month)

2 = occasionally (at least once a month)

3 = regularly (at least once a week)

4 = often (three or more days per week)

5 = constantly (every day).

Finally, indicate the severity of your symptoms on a scale of one to five where one is very mild and five is very severe.

Brain Fog Profile

Domain	Yes / No	Frequency	Severity
Executive function			
Attention			
Processing speed			
Learning and memory			
Language			
Visuo-spatial Processing			
Fatigue			

Congratulations, you made it!

Well done! You should be very proud and pleased. I really hope that you have enjoyed the journey so far. Day thirty is for celebrating and for assessing the progress that you have made, as well as for determining what has worked and what hasn't. Have a look at your progress and your successes, your new brain-healthy habits, but also look at the things that didn't quite work out and see whether you can identify why.

The hard work is done; many of your brain-healthy behaviours are now habits. You have laid the groundwork and embedded some really solid brain-healthy habits that you can to continue to implement and improve on. For now, you can bask in the glow of a job well done and enjoy a fog-free future of thinking faster, sharper, better.

Epilogue

I'd like to close by offering some final thoughts about what the future might hold for those of us affected by brain fog. It is appropriate that brain fog is not listed on the International Classification of Diseases (ICD-10) because it is not a disease or a disorder. But that doesn't mean that it's not real. Brain fog is very real; it is a symptom or a sign that something is amiss, just like a cough. The key to progress for those who experience brain fog is for doctors to accept this and to endeavour to determine what is driving the brain fog just as they would aim to ascertain whether the patient's cough is a sign or symptom of asthma, an infection, pneumonia or an allergy, for example. A good start would be for medical students to learn about brain fog during their training. You can also play a role in bringing about change by persisting with your doctor, asking them to work with you to find the underlying cause/s of your symptoms.

I am hopeful that the medical profession will start to pay more attention to brain fog and the significant impact that it can have on our lives. I think that we are already seeing moves in that direction, with some researchers and clinicians taking brain fog symptoms very seriously when they are experienced in the context of depression and multiple sclerosis. I am hopeful that this will become more commonplace.

Another concern is that some people don't even realise that they have brain fog. They put their cognitive dysfunction down to ageing and don't realise that brain fog is something that could be reversed quickly through lifestyle changes. We need more education and public awareness about brain health in general and we need to bust the myth that cognitive decline is a normal part of ageing.

I can't help but think – and I could be wrong – that the fact that more women than men are affected by both brain fog and many of the conditions that underlie it, is part of the reason why little progress has been made in finding cures and treatments. Women have long suffered and continue to suffer as a consequence of gender bias in both health research and healthcare. Most of the medical knowledge that exists today is based on human and animal research that excluded women, despite the fact that men and women differ at a cellular level in ways that mean that diseases and treatments may affect women and men differently.

A healthy brain needs a healthy cardiovascular system. Cardiovascular disease, the number one cause of death in women in the United States, affects women differently than men in terms of symptoms, risk factors and outcomes. Despite this, only a third of the people who take part in cardiovascular disease clinical trials are women. While this is a step up from the male-only studies of the past we still have a long way to go. Thankfully, more and more research funders are insisting that research studies are designed to take account of differences in sex and gender.

Ignoring differences between men and women in health research has had devastating and fatal consequences for women because of the assumption that treatments that work for men would work equally for women. The case of prescribing aspirin to prevent heart failure illustrates the situation very well. Early studies involving only men showed aspirin's protective effects. In 1993, the National Institute of Health mandated that women be included in any government health research to address the historic gender bias. To fill this historical gap, a separate women-only study on aspirin was carried out which failed to confirm the protective effect in women. In fact, when the data from multiple studies involving men and women were looked at, it emerged that while aspirin reduced the risk of heart attack but not stroke in men, it had the opposite effect in women, reducing risk of stroke but not heart attack.

We need to acknowledge the differences between men and women. Equality in health is not about treating people the same irrespective of their sex or gender but rather acknowledging differences where they exist to ensure that people get the best treatment and attain the best outcomes irrespective of sex or gender. Research into brain fog and conditions that underlie it has been scattered and lacking in focus. More investment and focus are needed to increase our understanding of this debilitating phenomenon that so disproportionately affects women.

When it comes to healthcare, women and men are not treated equally. Medical professionals behave differently towards women than men in terms of assessment, diagnosis, referral and treatment. Women are more likely to be misdiagnosed than men. A study that looked at 770 diseases found that, on average, women were diagnosed four years later than men. Mis-diagnosis and delayed diagnosis happen frequently in autoimmune diseases, which affect three times more women than men.

Even when women present with similar health problems to men, women are likely to receive a lower quality of care than men. It's highly unlikely that this is intentional. It's far more likely to be a result of uncon-scious gender biases or stereotypical views by medical professionals that are broadly based on two misconceptions – that women and men are physiologically the same or a failure to acknowledge the differences that actually do exist between women and men.

It could be that doctors take women's symptoms less seriously than men's. Maybe doctors don't understand or fail to take account of the fact that women experience symptoms differently to men. Or perhaps doctors attribute their female patients' symptoms to emotional rather than physiological causes. This could be due to the difference in the way males and females talk about their symptoms. Women tend to tell a story and talk about their symptoms in a personal way, while men tend to relay their symptoms in a more straightforward, factual way. I think these issues can become even more difficult when talking about cognitive symptoms because we (and I include both medical profes-sionals and patients in that 'we') have so little knowledge of brain and cognitive functioning. Plus I'm not convinced that doctors see problems with learning, memory, attention, executive function, language etc. as within their medical remit.

To improve assessment, diagnosis and treatment, doctors could learn to hear and interpret women's stories as they naturally tell them; alternatively, woman can decide to be more factual when presenting their symptoms. A bit of both is likely to produce the best results. For now, let's focus on the option we have control over – how we present our symptoms. Having read this book you are armed with knowledge about yourself, your symptoms, your brain and your brain fog. You have created a brain fog profile that pinpoints your specific symptoms; you have collected invaluable data from your logs and diaries about your symptoms and other factors, and you have taken note of pertinent symptoms that may help point doctors towards any potential underlying conditions. Presenting this information to your doctor in summary, together with your personal story of how your life has been impacted, should increase the likelihood that you will be heard and taken seriously. Hopefully this approach will improve the assessment, diagnosis and treatment that you receive. Be sure the doctor understands your story, don't let them cut you short, continue after the doctor's interruption, be persistent. When doctors ask 'yes'/'no' questions feel free to elaborate. If something doesn't feel right, speak up. If a diagnosis doesn't make sense to you discuss it further with your doctor. It's likely there are a list of possible diagnoses. Speaking up is critical; if you are not being heard I'd advise switching to a doctor who listens, understands medical differences and treats women with respect.

Knowledge is power. The more data that is collected from women living with brain fog, together with greater effort, resources and research focused on understanding brain fog, the greater our chances of preventing and treating the symptoms. I would like to see clinicians in general increase their understanding of brain health, brain fog and brain function. Whatever a clinician's particular speciality, the brain will always be involved.

At time of writing, COVID-19 has infected millions of people and claimed hundreds of thousands of lives across the globe. I would be remiss not to mention my concerns about the possible long-term effects on brain function. Although respiratory symptoms are most commonly associated with infection and death, there are increasing reports of brain and nervous system involvement. Neurological complications of COVID-19 reported to date include but are not limited to: stroke, inflammation of the membranes surrounding the brain and spinal cord and inflammation of the brain itself (meningoencephalitis), encephalopathy (brain damage and brain malfunction), death of brain tissue and micro bleeds in the brain. It's not known yet how the brain complications occur but prime suspects include either individually or in combination: direct injury from the virus, the effects of sepsis, low oxygen levels, high temperature, blood clots, hyperinflammation or inflammatory or immune disorders that occur in parallel with COVID-19 infection or post infection.

The main focus at present is on vaccinating and saving lives with outcomes only reported in terms of cases, deaths and recoveries. We need to move towards more nuanced reporting of outcomes that acknowledge, record and treat the long-term effects of infection. Communities of COVID-19 survivors experiencing long-term effects are springing up online. People join to share their ongoing symptoms, to find support among those also affected and also to seek action from government to address their plight. These 'Long COVID' communities are comprised of COVID-19 survivors, those with initially mild symptoms and undiagnosed individuals who suspect they had COVID-19 but couldn't access testing for various reasons. Anecdotal symptoms reported by the Long COVID community, online and in media interviews, commonly include brain fog. Survivors mention ongoing fatigue, pain, memory loss, difficulties focusing, concentrating or paying attention, language issues and generally feeling unwell or under par.

I am also concerned about the impact on brain function of the measures taken to prevent the spread of the virus, including lockdown, as well as the ongoing stress of living through a pandemic. Potential long-term effects in both non-infected and infected populations include post-traumatic stress disorder, depression, anxiety, poorly managed stress, insomnia, excess alcohol consumption and unhealthy lifestyle choices, all of which can lead to brain fog. The good news is that all of the information contained in this book is relevant to anyone who experiences brain fog irrespective of the underlying cause or precipitating factor/s.

The face of healthcare is changing at a rapid pace. New possibilities are emerging all the time. Technological and scientific advances, genome sequencing, data and informatics are being harnessed to make personalised care a reality. I am hopeful that as personalised medicine becomes mainstream it will accelerate progress in ways that will benefit people living with brain fog. While the knowledge gained from traditional research that focused mainly on males has taken decades to amass, big data analytics have the capacity to tap into the massive volume of clinically relevant but complex healthcare data on both males and females stored across different systems by healthcare organisations. Big data analytics could help to identify causes and risk factors and aid diagnosis and treatment. For example, hospital records, doctors' records, patient self-reports and even existing research literature, when pulled together to probe the right questions, could offer insights and reveal trends or patterns that could lead to greater understanding of brain fog or the hormonal fluctuations and medical conditions that can underlie it. Big data analytics also has the potential to inform diagnostics and treatment or support doctors to make more accurate diagnoses that take account of differences between men and women for example.

When personalised medicine is embedded in mainstream medicine, we may see more effective, tailored treatments based on a patient's personal profile, including their clinical history, their lifestyle and even their DNA. There is also potential for progress by using artificial intelligence; for example, to carry out digital diagnosis free from human error or biases. Of course, huge advances are being made in the field of genetics and, given the tendency for many of the conditions underlying brain fog to run in families, progress might be possible through DNA testing and possibly even gene editing. There is also potential to use AI to augment cognitive function when brain fog strikes.

I am passionate about raising awareness of the importance of brain health and really believe that if we could get people to look after their brain health as routinely as they look after their teeth, we would see a huge reduction in the incidence of brain fog together with a decrease in the severity of symptoms in those who remain affected. I would also like to see more people openly discussing brain fog and I would particularly like to hear more men talking about brain fog either in terms of their own experience or as advocates for the women affected.

Most of all, I hope that this book has helped you to beat brain fog. If it has please, please, do let me know; you can email me at info@superbrain.ie. And please do share your stories with others. We are all in this together and by sharing our experiences and our solutions we can change our collective future.

Symptoms

Use the next page to record any symptoms that you are experiencing. Presenting this information to your doctor in a succinct, structured and factual way may help with diagnosis and treatment. Using the information from your brain fog profile, make a note of the frequency and severity of your brain fog symptoms here. For example:

> *'I experience severe problems with memory and my ability to learn new things daily. For example, I have difficulty recalling the content of a meeting at work and this is interfering with my ability to do my job. In addition, I am finding that I can no longer perform tasks in my head. For example, I used to be able to figure out staff rosters in my head but now I have to write the information down and manipulate it on paper.*

> *'I also often have mild issues with language, at least three days a week. For example, I struggle to find the right word for things. I can cope at home by gesticulating and my family are pretty good at intuiting what I mean. It's a different story at work where it is incredibly embarrassing to endure blank faces and silence during what feels like an interminable pause when I go completely blank mid-sentence at a team meeting.'*

Symptoms

Glossary

1   **Cognition (cognitive function):** a group of mental processes that include attention, memory, producing and understanding language, learning, reasoning, problem-solving and decision-making.

2   **Perception (perceiving):** the process or outcome of becoming aware of objects, events and relationships through the senses. Includes observing, recognising and discriminating. Perception allows us to organise and interpret sensory information, transform the sensory information into useful knowledge and act in a coordinated fashion.

3   **Inhibitory control:** the ability to suppress interfering information or previously activated cognitive processes in order to focus attention on the relevant task requirements.

4   **Working memory:** refers to a system with limited capacity that can briefly store and manipulating information involved in the performance of complex cognitive tasks such as reasoning, comprehension and certain types of learning.

5   **Cognitive flexibility:** the ability to adapt behaviours in response to changes in the environment.

6   **Semantic memory:** memory for facts, general knowledge, words, numbers not related to personal experience. Semantic memory underlies processes such as recognising objects and using language.

7   **Reasonable accommodations:** effective and practical changes that an employer is required to put in place to enable a person with a disability to carry out their work on an equal footing with others. Reasonable accommodations take a variety of forms and can include flexible working arrangements, assistive technology or an adaptation of the physical workplace.

8   **Cytokines:** a group of proteins secreted by cells of the immune system that act as chemical messengers.

9   **Pathogen:** a tiny living organism that causes diseases to its host.

10 **Microbe:** a tiny living thing too small to be seen by the naked eye. Microbes are everywhere and millions of microbes call the human body home. Some microbes make us sick and others are essential for our health. The most common types are bacteria, viruses and fungi.

11 **Microbiota:** the human microbiota is made up of trillions of microbes. The biggest population reside in the gut although they also inhabit human skin and genitals. Microbial cells and their genetic material, the microbiome, live within humans from birth.

12   **Genes:** chromosomes hold the recipe for making a human and other living things. Found in the nucleus of every cell, chromosomes are made from strands of DNA. Segments of DNA are called genes. These genes are essentially the ingredients for the 'how to make a human' recipe. Each gene adds a specific protein to the recipe. Proteins build, regulate and maintain your body.

13   **Common endocrine-disrupting chemicals (ECDs):** DDT, Chlorpyrifos, Atrazine, 2, 4-D, Glyphosate, Lead, Phthalates, Cadmium, Bisphenol A (BPA), Phthalates, Phenol, Polychlorinated biphenyls (PCBs) and Dioxins, Brominated Flame Retardants, PCBs, Phthalates, Parabeans, UV Filters, Triclosan and Perfluorochemicals.

14   **BPA-free:** BPA (bisphenol A) is an industrial chemical used to make certain plastics including polycarbonate plastics and epoxy resins. The former is often used in containers that store food and drinks including water bottles. While the latter are used to coat the inside of cans, bottle tops and water supply lines. Research shows that BPA from containers can seep into food and drinks. BPA has oestrogenic activity, linking it to endocrine disease and an increased risk of endocrine-related cancers.

15   **BHPF:** a BPA substitute called flurene-9-bisphenol used in 'BPA-free' plastics. Some research suggests that BHPF has anti-oestrogenic activity and more research is required to determine the toxicological effects of BHPF on health.

16   **Genetic code:** the set of rules by which information encoded in genetic material (DNA or RNA sequences) is translated into proteins by living cells.

17   **Oxidative stress:** oxidative stress occurs when there is an imbalance between the production of free radicals and the ability of the body to counteract or detoxify their harmful effects through neutralisation by antioxidants. Oxidative stress can lead to heart and blood vessel disorders, heart failure, heart attack and neurodegenerative diseases including Parkinson's disease and Alzheimer's disease.

18   **Gluten ataxia:** gluten is a protein found in wheat, barley and rye. Ataxia refers to a group of neurological symptoms that affect speech, coordination and balance. When an individual with gluten sensitivity eats gluten, their immune system produces antibodies that can attack the balance centres in the brain, leading to ataxia.

19   **Peripheral neuropathy:** develops when nerves in the hands, arms, feet or legs are damaged, resulting in weakness, numbness and pain.

20   **Prophylactic:** a medicine intended to prevent disease or, in this instance, occurrence of migraine.

21   **Endocannabinoid:** the endocannabinoid system (ECS) is a cell signalling system involved in sleep, mood, appetite and memory. Cannabinoids are active compounds found in cannabis. Endocannabinoids are similar to cannabinoids but produced by your body. The ECS is active in your body even if you don't consume cannabis. There are two main receptors: one type found in the CNS and one type found in the PNS. Results depends on the location of the receptor and which endocannabinoids bind to it. For example, binding to one type in a spinal nerve to relieve pain, or in your immune cells to signal that your body is experiencing inflammation.

22   **Biofilm:** a collection of microbial cells enclosed in an extracellular substance. The slimy build-up of bacteria that forms on the surfaces of teeth called dental plaque is an example of a biofilm.

23 Recommended hours of sleep per day:

Age	Recommended range per 24 hours
65+	7 to 8 hours
18 to 64	7 to 9 hours
14 to 17	8 to 10 hours
6 to 13	9 to 11 hours
3 to 5	10 to 13 hours
1 to 2	11 to 14 hours
4 to 11 months	12 to 15 hours
0 to 3 months	14 to 17 hours

24 **Noradrenaline:** a hormone and a neurotransmitter involved in mobilising the brain and body for action.

25 **Dopamine:** a neurotransmitter involved in multiple functions including reward, pleasure and movement.

26 **Antioxidant:** a substance, such as vitamin E, vitamin C, or beta-carotene, thought to protect body cells from the damaging effects of oxidation.

Bibliography

All quotes from Sun Tzu taken from Tzu, Sun (1910). *The Art of War*, translated by Lionel Giles

Chapter 1 – Know the Enemy: Brain Fog

Diamond, A., (2013). Executive functions. *Annual Reviews Psychology.* 64: 135–168, doi 10.1146/annurev-psych-113011-14375

Logue, S.F., Gould, T.J., (2013). The Neural and Genetic Basis of Executive Function: Attention, Cognitive Flexibility, and Response Inhibition. 0: 45–54. doi: 10.1016/j. pbb.2013.08.007

Chapter 3 – Know Yourself: Your Brain

Anderson, S.C., Cryan, J.F., and Dinan, T., (2019). The Psychobiotic Revolution; *National Geographic*

Chapter 4 – Know Yourself: Your Hormones

Ali S. A., Begum, T., and Reza, F., (2018). Hormonal influences on cognitive function. *Malays J Med Sci.* 25(4): 31–41. https://doi.org/10.21315/mjms2018.25.4.3

Celec, P., Ostatnikova, D., and Hodosay, J., (2015). On the effects of testosterone on brain behavioural functions. *Frontiers in Neuroscience,* 9: 12. doi: 10.3389/fnins.2015.00012

Chen, H., Yang, Y.M., Han, R., and Nobel, M., (2013). MEK 1/2 Inhibition Suppresses Tamoxifen Toxity on CNS Glial Progenitor Cells. *Journal of Neuroscience.* 33(38): 15069–15074. doi: https://doi.org/10.1523/JNEUROSCI.2729-13.2013

Glaser, R., and Dimitrakakis, C., (2013). Testosterone therapy in women: myths and misconceptions. *Maturitas.* 74: 230–234

Gore, A.C., Crews, D., Doan, L.L., La Merrill, M., Patisaul, D.H., and Zota, A., (2014). Introduction to Endocrine Disrupting Chemicals (EDCs) A Guide for Public Interest Organisations and Policy-makers. Published by the Endocrine Society and IPEN

Hertel, J., Konig, J., Homuth, G., et al., (2017). Evidence for Stress-like Alterations in the HPA-Axis in Women Taking Oral Contraceptives. *Scientific Reports.* 1:14111. doi:10.1038/s41598-017-13927-7

Hill, S., (2019). *This is Your Brain on Birth Control.* Orion Spring

Kabir, R., Rahman, M., and Rahman, I., (2015). A review on endocrine disruptors and their possible impacts on human health. *Environmental Toxicology and Pharmacology.* 40: 241–258

McKay, S., (2018). *Demystifying the Female Brain.* Orion Spring

McEwen, B.S., and Alves, S.E., (1999). Estrogen Actions in the Central Nervous System. *Endocrine Reviews.* 20(3): 279–307

Zárate S., Stevnsner, T., Gredilla R., (2017). Role of Estrogen and Other Sex Hormones in Brain Aging. Neuroprotection and DNA Repair. *Frontiers in Aging Neuroscience.* 9: 430. doi:10.3389/fnagi.2017.00430

Chapter 5 – Know Yourself: Your Defences

Borsook, D., (2012), A Future without Chronic Pain: Neuroscience and Clinical Research. *Cerebrum.* 7

Cohen, E., (2004). My self as an other: on autoimmunity and 'other' paradoxes. *Medical Humanities.* 30: 7–11

Crocker, H., Jenkinson, C., and Peters, M., (2018). Quality of life in coeliac disease: qualitative interviews to develop candidate items for the Coeliac Disease Assessment Questionnaire. *Patient Related Outcome Measures.* 9: 211–220, doi: 10.2147/PROM. S149238

Dantzer, R., O'Connor, J.C., Freund, G.G., Johnson, R.W., and Kelley, K.W., (2008). From inflammation to sickness and depression: when the immune system subjugates the brain. *Nature reviews. Neuroscience.* 9(1): 46–56. doi:10.1038/nrn2297

Mackay, M., (2015). Lupus brain fog: a biologic perspective on cognitive impairment, depression, and fatigue in systemic lupus erythematosus. *Immunol Res.* 63: 26–37. doi: 10.1007/s12026-015-8716-3

Moriarty, O., McGuire, B.E., and Finn, D.P., (2011). The effect of pain on cognitive function: a review of clinical and preclinical research. *Prog Neurobiol.* 93(3): 385–404. doi: 10.1016/j.pneurobio.2011.01.002

Nuñez, F.P., Maraver, M.J., and Colzato, L.S., (2019). Sex Hormones as Cognitive Enhancers? *Neuro Endocrinology Letters.* 23 Suppl., 4: 67–77

Ocon, A.J., (2013). Caught in the thickness of brain fog: exploring the cognitive symptoms of Chronic Fatigue Syndrome. *Frontiers in Physiology.* 2: 63. doi: 10.3389/fphys.2013.00063

Orchard, T.S., Gaudier-Diaz, M.M., Weinhold, K.R., and Courtney DeVries, A., (2017). Clearing the fog: a review of the effects of dietary omega-3 fatty acids and added sugars on chemotherapy-induced cognitive deficits. *Breast cancer research and treatment.* 161(3): 391–398. https://doi.org/10.1007/s10549-016-4073-8

Pahwa, R., Singh, A., and Jialal, I., Chronic Inflammation. [Updated 2019 Dec 13]. In: StatPearls [Internet]. Treasure Island (FL): StatPearls Publishing; 2019 Jan. Available from: https://www.ncbi.nlm.nih.gov/books/NBK493173

Walker, K.A., Hoogeveen, R.C., Folsom, A.R., Ballantyne, C.M., Knopman, D.S., Windham, B.G., Jack, C.R., and Gottesman, R.F., (2017). Midlife systemic inflammatory markers are associated with late-life brain volume. *Neurology.* doi: 10.1212/WNL.0000000000004688

Yelland, G.W., (2017). Gluten-induced cognitive impairment (brain fog) in coeliac disease. *Journal of Gasteroenterology and Hepatology.* 32, (Suppl. 1): 90–93. doi:10.1111/jgh.13706

Chapter 6 – Power: Brain Health

Brennan, S., (2019). *100 Days to a Younger Brain.* Orion Spring

Chapter 7 – Sleep

Eisenstein, M., (2013). Chronobiology: Stepping out of time. *Nature.* 497: S10-S12

Horne, J.A., and Östberg, O., (1976). A self-assessment questionnaire to determine morningness-eveningness in human circadian rhythms. *International Journal of Chronobiology.* 4: 97–110

Marquié, J., Tucker, P., Folkard, S., et al. (2015). Chronic effects of shift work on cognition: findings from the VISAT longitudinal study. *Occupational and Environmental Medicine.* 72: 258–264

Walker, M., (2017). *Why We Sleep.* Scribner

Chapter 8 – Stress

Kobassa, S.C., (1979). Stress, life events, personality and health: and inquiry into hardiness. *Journal of Personality and Social Psychology.* 42: 168–177

McKay, S., (2018). *Demystifying the Female Brain.* Orion Spring

Schmaal, L., et al., (2016). Subcortical brain alterations in major depressive disorder: findings from the ENIGMA Major Depressive Disorder working group. *Mol Psychiatry.* 21(6): 806–12

Chapter 9 – Exercise

Di Liegro, C.M., Schiera, G., Proia, P., and Di Liegro, I., (2019). Physical Activity and Brain Health. *Genes.* 10(9): 720. https://doi.org/10.3390/genes10090720

Northey, J.M., Cherbuin, N., Pumpa, K.L., et al., (2018). Exercise interventions for cognitive function in adults older than 50: a systematic review with meta-analysis. *British Journal of Sports Medicine.* 52: 154–160

Raichlen, D.A., and Alexander, G.E., (2020). Why Your Brain Needs Exercise. *Scientific American.* 322(1): 26–31

Chapter 10 – Nutrition

Carmona, R., (2014). *30 Days to a Better Brain.* Simon and Schuster

Dye, L., Boyle, N.B., Champ, C., and Lawton, C., (2017). The relationship between obesity and cognitive health and decline. *Proc Nutr Soc.* 76(4): 443–454. doi: 10.1017/S0029665117002014

Global Council on Brain Health, (2019). The Real Deal on Brain Health Supplements: GCBH Recommendations on Vitamins, Minerals, and Other Dietary Supplements. Available at www.GlobalCouncilOnBrainHealth.org. doi: https://doi.org/10.26419/pia.00094.001

Okereke, O.I., Rosner, B.A., Kim, D.H., et al., (2012). Dietary fat types and 4-year cognitive change in community-dwelling older women. doi.org/10.1002/ana.23593

Chapter 11 – 30-Day Plan

Duhigg, C., (2013). *The Power of Habit.* William Heinmann

Global Council on Brain Health, (2018). 'Brain-Food GCBH Recommendations on Nourishing Your Brain Health.' Available at: www.GlobalCouncilOnBrainHealth.org. https://doi.org/10.26419/pia.00019.001

Rubin, G., (2009). *The Happiness Project.* HarperCollins

Acknowledgements

If you're expecting a witty, entertaining declaration of thanks, you'll be disappointed. Despite reading how to write 'amazing acknowledgements' I still have nothing, nada, zero, zilch, nowt. In comparison, writing this book was a doddle. Mainly because Pippa Wright is an absolute dream to work with. Plus she's a dog-lover, a list-maker and a Gemini, what's not to like? Pippa, your edits were excellent, encouraging and exciting, they made my heart sing and my feet dance. Thank you for believing in me, I've really enjoyed making this book with you. We make a good team.

Speaking of teams, I want to thank Dizzy and Daisy for their loyalty. They doggedly sat beside me as I wrote every word. In fact, Dizzy frequently sprawled across my keyboard as she vied with my laptop for attention. These girls made me smile every day and demanded that I take restorative breaks to give them belly rubs and play ball. Oh the guilt for not mentioning my other dogs. Nuts, I know, but I also know that if I don't mention Scruffy and Kim, certain family members will be on my case for showing favouritism.

Speaking of families, mine is small but perfectly formed. Naff as it sounds, they are the centre of my world. Dave, I want to thank you for keeping the plates spinning while I wrote this book. I'd like to list everything that you did and do, but I won't because that would make me sound incredibly lazy. Gavin and Jamie, thanks for all the bits and bobs that you do for me, again no lists, see above. Darren, your medical insights have been invaluable. Caoimhe, thank you for making Darren happy.

Zoe King, you made me incredibly happy when you secured the publishing deal for this book. You are an amazing agent. I love your big picture thinking and am indebted to you for pushing me to put myself out there. Your confidence gives me courage. Rebecca Ritchie, I really appreciate your sound advice, patience and attentiveness while Zoe creates her own little masterpiece. Georgia Goodall, thank you for making the editing process a seamless, stress-free experience. To everyone at Orion Spring, it's been a really pleasant journey, here's to many more.

The final nod goes to you, Sharon Bowers, for your incredibly useful noodling and sage advice. You're up next.

Credits

The author and Orion Spring would like to thank everyone at Orion who worked on the publication of *Beating Brain Fog*.

Agent
Zoe King
Rebecca Ritchie

Editor
Pippa Wright

Copy-editor
Liz Marvin

Proofreader
Sue Lascelles

**Editorial
Management**
Georgia Goodall
Jane Hughes
Claire Boyle

Audio
Paul Stark
Amber Bates

Contracts
Anne Goddard
Paul Bulos
Jake Alderson

Design
Lucie Stericker
Joanna Ridley
Rabab Adams
Clare Sivell
Helen Ewing

Finance
Jennifer Muchan
Jasdip Nandra
Rabale Mustafa
Elizabeth Beaumont
Afeera Ahmed
Ibukun Ademefun
Sue Baker
Tom Costello

Production
Nicole Abel
Fiona McIntosh

Marketing
Jennifer Hope

Publicity
Elizabeth Allen

Sales
Jennifer Wilson
Victoria Laws
Esther Waters
Frances Doyle
Ben Goddard
Georgina Cutler
Jack Hallam
Ellie Kyrke-Smith
Inês Figueira
Barbara Ronan
Rachael Jones
Andrew Hally
Dominic Smith
Deborah Deyong
Lauren Buck
Maggy Park
Linda McGregor
Sinead White
Jemimah James
Jack Dennison
Nigel Andrews
Ian Williamson
Julia Benson
Declan Kyle

Robert Mackenzie
Megan Smith
Charlotte Clay
Rebecca Cobbold

Operations
Jo Jacobs
Helen Gibbs
Sharon Willis
Lucy Brem
Sneha Wharton
Steven Dennant
Lucy Olley
Rochelle Dowden-Lord
Isobel Sheene

Rights
Susan Howe
Richard King
Krystyna Kujawinska
Jessica Purdue
Louise Henderson

About the Author

Dr Sabina Brennan is a chartered health psychologist, neuroscientist, award-winning science communicator, author of the international best-seller *100 Days to a Younger Brain* and host of the critically-acclaimed *Super Brain* podcast.

Dr Brennan leads Brain Fit, a large-scale research study on brain health, lifestyle, genomics and dementia risk at Trinity College Dublin, Ireland's premier university.

Dr Brennan has been engaged as an advisor to governments and global businesses influencing policy and practice in the areas of brain health, ageing, dementia, migraine and multiple sclerosis. She also volunteers on scientific advisory boards and advocacy panels supporting charities, non-profits and NGOs.